The Food
BONDAGE

Making a Case for the Human Diet

Gregory Stypko

To Mom

Table of Contents

.

Introduction

What do you do when you realize that an official, widespread position on an issue affecting virtually *everybody* may be wrong? I am talking about the realization that the scientifically supported, government-backed nutritional policy is holding us back from living our optimally healthy lives. I came to this awareness upon discovering that the natural human way of eating is very different from the one to which we currently subscribe. It's so dissimilar that it doesn't even jibe with any of the alternative diets proposed to us so far. Yes, I know what natural human nutrition used to be. I neither guess nor suspect it; I know it. And I am astonished that our prototypical way of eating hasn't been publicized by now. It's one of those concepts that, once it really sinks in, makes perfect sense. For one thing, it immediately explains the variety of the diets that we pursue as well as their claims of effectiveness. And it perfectly fits the model of our ancestral, evolution-shaped way of eating.

When I first came to this conclusion, I instinctively questioned my judgment, since I couldn't believe, as obvious as it is to me, that this diet hasn't ever been evaluated or proposed as a viable eating alternative, at least to my knowledge. Instead, we as a society have officially promoted nutrition based on a millennia-old eating tradition.

Going against a long-standing official policy is never easy—especially in the current social climate, where anybody can have a voice through social media channels and our various internet platforms that are rife with quackery, half-truths, and outright falsehoods. In that environment, conspiracy theories abound, and the undermining of authorities has become quite popular. So, here I am amidst that confusing informational landscape, telling you that the official nutritional policy may not be best suited for us.

I think most of us already suspect that something is off in how this subject is treated today. However, we don't realize how significantly our current diet deviates from our natural one. According to experts, in addition to possibly being ill-advised, straying from the standard dietary course can be outright dangerous. But fortunately, not everybody agrees with the official line of thinking. There are nutritionists and doctors in unconventional dietary camps who strongly disagree with the orthodox dietary approach. Some of them recognize that the current high-carb, grain-based, three-meals-daily nutrition is not what it's cracked up to be. However, their persuasive power is minuscule because, despite their credentials, they constitute but a tiny fraction of the nutritional establishment. Their words are not heard outside the small community of diet experimenters. And thus, most of us are doomed to follow the official guidelines—no matter how badly they affect our quality of living.

My initial motivation to write this book was the frustration I experienced with my pesky food addictions, health problems, and inability to control my weight, as well as the fact that many other people around me were and are fighting the same unfair battle with food. When I started writing on this topic, I compared our food consumption to our ancestors'. The juxtaposition spurred the acknowledgment that I had never really stopped to appreciate the level of involvement required of them to survive. That, in turn, made me rethink my other idyllic preconceptions about their lifestyle. Finally, I came to understand that when we try to imagine the everyday routine of our predecessors, their dietary habits become obvious. These habits simply could not have been any different, because they were enforced by the reality of their circumstances. Similarly, our modern eating habits are imposed by the genetics we share with our predecessors and our modern nutritional environment.

Before I continue, let me tell you about myself. I am neither a medical practitioner nor a dietitian. I am an engineer. I hold a Master of Science degree in electronics and I have spent most of my professional life working as a software engineer. I am not qualified to tell anybody how and what they should eat, and that's not my intention. However, based on my research and analysis, I would like to demonstrate how we are evolutionarily adapted to nourish our bodies. And, since most of the experts are disinterested or unclear on the subject, I feel justified in presenting my view.

My fundamental problem with most experts' approach to nutrition is their disregard for the link between our optimal health and our genetic adaptation, which is obvious in my opinion. It seems that the starting point for nutritionists is the food we have at our disposal now and the eating tradition we have subscribed to for generations. That is the reason why, until now, we have not established an optimal human nutrition theory. Rather, we are presented with an array of diets, each conflicting with others and claiming to be the correct one. Those regimes, including the one that is currently recommended by the authorities, are based on seemingly solid scientific studies. They are based on research-backed books written by respected nutritional and medical professionals. And yet, despite or perhaps because of all the revelations popping up nowadays, we are perpetually stuck in the same dietary turmoil.

What is the reason for this confusion? My view on the subject is the following, in a nutshell: Our inability to zero in on the optimal human diet is due to our flawed approach to the subject. Namely, we are trying to draw conclusions from a fragmentary knowledge of enormously complex subjects. Multi-year population dietary studies are one example of those attempts. Another is our detailed research into the digestion and metabolism-related processes of the human body. In both cases, with the huge number of variables and unknowns, we are simply unable to make unambiguous determinations.

However, forming a detailed understanding of population studies and the super-complex life processes involved in human sustenance are not the only ways to gain insight into our optimal nutrition method. An alternative would be to consider how the environment and our instincts enforce a particular form of eating. And that is my approach to both subjects of this book: our food dependence in today's world and our optimal nutritional model.

While we are drowning in the vast amount of available information on diets and foods, there are fundamental questions that never get answered. One of those is: On what basis did we decide that starch-based food three times a day is best for us?

I haven't found a satisfactory response to that question. It seems to me that we have followed that particular dietary formula unquestioningly for generations. The decisions concerning our staple foods and the way they should be eaten were made for us thousands of years ago when our ancestors settled and started farming. They created a particular diet based merely on viable crops. That nutritional switch was radical because it changed their foods as well as the way they were eaten. If we agree that our nutrition before the farming revolution was the proper human diet, we have to acknowledge that our modern way of eating is... not the human diet.

Let me clarify: It is invented by us but is not natural to our species. And yet, we base our well-being on the prehistoric dietary construct that we back with modern science and medicine.

Am I the only one seeing a paradox here?

This book has a twofold purpose. The first is to expose our health and dietary dysfunction and point out the ways in which nutrition dominates our lives; in other words, why it's nearly impossible to escape overeating. The second is to present the real human diet and the role it could play in fixing our current health disaster.

The book is divided into three parts. The first shows the full extent of our nutritional anomaly and its impact on our quality of life. In this part, I will address our tacit agreement to treat our nutritional situation as an inevitability of civilizational progress. I will also discuss the shifting of public focus from failing nutritional standards to medication as the way to deal with the current health crisis.

The second part deals with the details of our multifaceted, unwholesome relationship with eating. Here, I will take a look at the current nutritional guidelines and consider the reasons for overeating, which include culture, cravings, addictions, and nutritional advice.

The third part of the book introduces our ancestral diet and shows its various implications. In this part, I will describe the fallacies we commit in our assumptions about the life of the hunter-gatherer and their optimal nutrition and longevity. Then I will analyze the critical differences between our diet and our predecessors', explaining why early human nutrition must have been structured in a specific way. I will offer an example of a consumption model following our natural eating pattern and present suggestions on how the authorities could approach long-overdue nutritional reform. Subsequently, I will present my personal dietary struggles, including my transition to the human diet. I will conclude with the argument for the human diet as the best solution for our current failing food consumption model.

I am glad to have you explore this important subject with me.

Part One

Chapter One

Dystopia

Despite spectacular progress in many areas, our country, together with the rest of the industrialized world, suffers a permanent health crisis caused by the improper nourishment of its citizens. Notwithstanding longer life expectancy, the quality of life of the majority of U.S. citizens is appalling. Overweight, with many of us also depressed and relying heavily on pharmaceuticals, we are stuck in an unhealthy nutritional lifestyle as captives of the official food policy.

One doesn't have to look far to confirm the magnitude of our nutritional health crisis. Here is the data from the government's 2015-2020 Dietary Guidelines:[1]

About half of all American adults—117 million individuals— have one or more preventable chronic diseases, many of which are related to poor quality eating patterns and physical

---

[1] U.S. Department of Health and Human Services and U.S. Department of Agriculture. **"2015–2020 Dietary Guidelines for Americans."**8th Edition. Last modified December 2015.Accessed March 10, 2018. **https://health.gov/dietaryguidelines/2015/guidelines/**.

inactivity. These include cardiovascular disease, high blood pressure, type 2 diabetes, some cancers, and poor bone health. More than two-thirds of adults and nearly one-third of children and youth are overweight or obese. These high rates of overweight and obesity and chronic disease have persisted for more than two decades and come not only with increased health risks but also at a high cost. In 2008, the medical costs associated with obesity were estimated to be $147 billion. In 2012, the total estimated cost of diagnosed diabetes was $245 billion including $176 billion in direct medical costs and $69 billion in decreased productivity.

The latest statistics are nothing new. For years, they have been showing the same ominous trend. We are getting bigger, and we are getting sicker. And, without minimizing the impact of physical inactivity, poor nutrition is the principal cause of that predicament. That situation exists despite the decades-long remedial educational effort by the government. The apparent failure of the current strategy of "gentle persuasion" should raise questions about the justification of its continuation in its current form.

After all, nearly everybody is aware of the nutritional guidelines. We've heard about the margarine recommendations, butter warnings, and various food pyramids and plates. One would think that by now everyone realizes the dangerous consequences of unhealthy eating, and yet, the majority of the population continues to follow risky eating patterns.

What is the cause of that seemingly irrational behavior? Why is it impossible to convince people to adhere to the recommended diet? Is there any way other than persuasion to correct this situation? These questions beg to be discussed on a national forum, as they're keys to resolving the current health disaster.

Over the years, we've been able to overcome a multitude of health challenges, including the high infant mortality rate and scourges like polio, tuberculosis, and most recently HIV.

However, something as straightforward as altering eating habits seems like a hopeless proposition. Why is it such a difficult problem to solve? After all, we live in times of extraordinary technological advancement. We are seeing the beginning of commercial space exploration, self-driving cars, virtual reality, and imminent artificial intelligence. Twenty-first-century progress permeates almost every aspect of our lives—except nutrition. Is it because nutrition has a special status that can't be encroached on? It certainly looks that way, for whatever reason. We can look at every other civilizational impediment in a practical way. For example, we've been able to completely change our methods of transportation, telecommunication, and interaction with each other through social media. Likewise, we successfully tamed common vices like the widespread use of alcohol and tobacco. Food, however, presents a special case. It appears that, beyond persuasion, we are incapable of effectively mounting the fight against bad nourishment. Why?

Perhaps there is something wrong with the advice we are getting from the government and its affiliated authorities in this field. In fact, many doubt the wisdom of the official recommendations, believing that the prescribed steady high-carbohydrate, low-fat diet is more of an impediment than a feasible dietary proposition. The science doesn't seem to help in that respect, as many nutritional studies contradict themselves. They indicate various macronutrient ratios as the path to maintaining a healthy weight. As a result, we have entrenched camps throwing their support behind the high-carbohydrate diets on the one side and the low-carbohydrate ones on the other. Who's right? Is it possible that they are all right and wrong at the same time? This seemingly contradictory hypothesis will be explored in the subsequent chapters. Whatever is the reason for their failure, the current recommendations don't work for the majority of Americans. With that in mind, it's important to acknowledge that the available nutritional advice is not the only factor influencing consumption. There is also the availability of foods and their price structure. That is where the authorities come in again. While food production and sales are governed by market forces, the government is indirectly shaping our diet through farming subsidies. The resulting artificial price structure encourages us to consume more grains, which are offered inexpensively, courtesy of the incentives.

While there are certainly more factors shaping our eating pattern, the two significant ones—official nutritional advice and food pricing structure—are the purview of the government. That makes the powers that be largely responsible for our current dietary mayhem.

Is there anything that we can do as citizens to influence a change? Certainly; we can't just give up. We shouldn't be satisfied with the current situation, in which almost three-quarters of us are overweight or obese and prone to many dangerous illnesses. Neither should we regard as normal our typical modern cityscape, dominated by junk food places conveniently interspaced with pharmacies.

We should realize that while the authorities pay lip service to change our diet, they don't seriously attempt to improve it. Contrary to the pundits' implications, we (the great majority) are not gluttons. Rather, it's hard for us to make rational nutritional decisions in the current environment. We are being flooded with tempting food offerings bolstered by unrestrained, aggressive advertising. Consumers are caught between food industry marketing and governmental persuasion.

Obviously, the two influences have different effectiveness. While the free market forces are very capable of making us fat, governmental efforts seem to be utterly inept. Let's consider both tactics.

On the one hand, we have professionally-managed marketing campaigns. They depict happy people in comfortable social situations enjoying their inexpensive sodas, snacks, pizzas, and burgers. Their power of persuasion is bolstered by the fact that the super-caloric food they promote is, in fact, deliciously addictive.

On the other hand, we have our fractured understanding of nutrition and the authorities' timid "this might be bad for you" message buried in government websites.

In our free market world, food is a commodity like any other and profit is king. Thus, what counts in the end is to sell the maximum quantity of the most profitable goods. Those strategies work well for the food industry—just look at the giants of the fast food and soda industry. Or for that matter, the pharmaceutical industry. Due to our widespread, nutritionally impeded health issues, we've built up large pharmaceutical corporations which happily provide us with a plentitude of remedies for hypertension, diabetes, high cholesterol, and even erectile dysfunction. As good as it is for business, what are the consequences? How does this state of affairs affect our individual lives? Couldn't it be argued that we are way too dependent on deliciously toxic meals and powerful, pricey pharmaceuticals? And finally, does the unrestrained free market approach make sense?

Following that line of thought, there are some fundamental questions that need to be answered. Isn't highly caloric food addictive? Can we rely on ourselves to make correct nutritional choices cool-headedly? How does our diet compare to the one that our bodies have evolved to eat? We don't ask these questions because we have gotten used to the sustenance available to us. In addition to the powerful physiological attraction of our junk foods, we associate them with happy moments. Also, we are being conditioned to favor the not-so-healthy foods socially, starting in early childhood. That training goes back quite a long time; previous generations were also subjected to the temptation of these super-caloric delights. But it's only relatively recently that the foods which in excess make us sick have become mass-produced, mass-marketed, and cheap.

Given that, our self-destructive nutritional choices are not shocking at all. One may even say our strong preference for caloric "bombs" is reasonable, as they are inexpensive, addictive, omnipresent, and socially accepted.

While the health crisis has settled permanently into our reality, the ongoing debate focuses mostly on the issue of mandatory universal healthcare. Among the heated arguments about its legitimacy, nobody addresses the elephant in the room: the improper nutrition of our population.

While bickering about the health care system, we accept the appalling health situation itself. We implicitly agree with the idea that our nourishment predicament is a behavioral problem caused by the common lack of self-control. We don't explore the addictive nature of the highly caloric foods that dominate our supermarkets. Hence, the conclusion is that the obesity crisis is an unavoidable result of our civilizational progress, and we the citizens are left to cope on an individual level since the government has done all it can to resolve the problem. Really?

Here is how the authorities are trying to solve the healthcare crisis.

On the prevention front, they offer guidelines for healthy nutrition and physical activity. To address health problems arising from diet-induced chronic conditions, they back powerful medications which regulate cholesterol, blood pressure, insulin level, and so on. Our healthcare specialists are making great progress in prolonging cancer patients' lives; however, we as a society are not faring as well with Alzheimer's disease, dementia, and other mental conditions which may be affected by nutrition.

As to healthcare: We keep restructuring its management in attempts to mitigate the consequences of the increased demand for medical services and costly treatments.

Curiously, the authorities gloss over the cause of the problem— the nutritional dystopia. The main thrust of the government's remedial action is directed toward fixing healthcare.

Thus, on the margin of the healthcare dispute, the issue of nutrition is being regarded as an inevitable nuisance.

As we are painfully aware, the government's approach to solving both problems has proven ineffective. Despite the years of publishing nutritional advice and countless healthcare reorganizations, the healthcare crisis has worsened. The discussion about health insurance is a red herring; it shifts the focus from the source of the problem, nutrition, to its consequence, the growing expenses of healthcare.

At the risk of overstating the obvious, I assert that the only sensible approach is to seriously address the root of the crisis—our improper diet. The first step to fixing it is the admission that our choice of foods is different from most other practical decisions we make. The second is the realization that subsidizing cheap grain production while leaving the food supply at the mercy of market forces is a recipe for disaster.

Our collective health situation is pretty dire. As things stand right now, there are millions of people suffering from heart conditions, dementia, depression, diabetes, cancers, and many other diet-triggered illnesses. Over many years, those people have been eating themselves into horrible health problems. It's easy to label them as careless or ignorant. However, they are neither. They are just more susceptible to the powerful lure of super-caloric food. Their curse is their primal adaptation to times of food scarcity and consequent maladaptation to times of constant plentitude. If the cause of their affliction were a virus, we all would be up in arms trying to combat the vicious microbe. However, when the condition is "preventable," we rationalize our quasi-neutral attitude. We persuade ourselves that they are victims of their unhealthy choices, and their fate is just the price they have to pay.

It's not that we are unsympathetic. Naturally, as a society, we make sure that we all survive as long as possible, despite astronomical costs. In our compassion, we go even farther: We provide our nutritional invalids with lots of special parking spaces, wheelchair ramps, heart defibrillators, and even drivable shopping carts. It's a good thing that we do that; however, it points to the enormous scale of the problem. When we see those disabled in public places, we've got to realize that they are just the tip of the iceberg. A vast majority of them are invisible to us as they spend their lives shut in their homes or in specialized care institutions with family or caretakers watching over them. The situation with so many people not being able to function independently in times of peace is at absurd levels. It evokes accounts of post-war nations—except, while many soldiers and civilians suffer physical and psychological injuries due to real bullets, grenades, shrapnel, bombs, and other horrors of war, we now have people hurting because they overconsume innocent-looking calorie bombs.

One of the goals of this book is to present the proper human diet and push for nutritional reform. Not just a correction to bring us in line with those countries faring better nutritionally, but a significant change to the food structure and the way we consume. A transformation like this will not be painless, as it will require rethinking our traditional celebratory approach to eating. However, living in the twenty-first century, we should be ready to shake off the emotional bond that we associate with nutrition. We have to look at eating comprehensively and dispassionately, as the best way of fueling our bodies. We must start with a clean slate. The cornerstone of the reform has to be the human evolutionary adaptation—instead of what's traditional, convenient, tasty, or inexpensive to produce. Those four reasons have served us mixed results for centuries and have finally brought us to where we are today. We are stuck in a primal cravings-driven, tradition-formed, and market-controlled food consumption pattern. While that model can be improved, it can't get us to the best nutrition formula possible.

As we are having a fresh look at our nourishment, we ought to ask ourselves this question: Is our traditional, millennia-old farming menu optimally healthy? Certainly not. However, due to our omnivorous adaptability, we have been able to cope, many of us living into our eighties and the luckiest of us even into their hundreds. Nevertheless, that medicine-sustained life extension comes at the cost of severely diminished quality of life. Taking a dietary leap forward, we should aim high. We should focus on our predispositions instead of trying to fit our eating style between tradition and the market forces, and while doing that, we should also rethink our food production and pricing structure.

We should rewind our eating practices about ten thousand years, to the period before farming—that is, to the extended period that formed our primal dietary adaptation. At the same time, we should not equate that optimal way of eating with the trendy hunter-gatherer or Paleo diets.

We have to keep in mind that for practical reasons, we can't return to the hunter-gatherer style of eating, as we function in an entirely altered world now. Our level and pattern of activities are different, and so are the foods that we have at our disposal. However, we can use certain aspects of our modern status quo to our advantage and thereby do much better than our almost anatomically identical Stone Age ancestors. We have a chance to emulate their nutrition where it matters and dovetail it with modern agriculture and food production methods, nutrition research, and medicine. Instead of overtaxing our health practitioners, we should focus on prevention of diet-caused illness in a big way; we should acknowledge as inescapable fact that diet is the best remedy. And, despite our medical prowess, the change of eating habits is as close to a "miracle cure" as we can get to. From today's point of view, that cure could surpass the achievements of today's remedial medicine. It could prevent most of today's common and rare ailments. At the same time, it would entirely refocus our medical science on extending lifespan beyond our genetic limits. Also, a more significant emphasis could be placed on the monitoring of the influence of environmental toxicity on our health.

The relevant question at this juncture may be: Can we really expect such huge changes from merely improving our nutrition? The key to anticipating the results of the proposed diet shift is the realization that there is enormous health improvement potential even in revising only certain aspects of our current diet. We can look at Japan to see that this is a quite realistic hypothesis. The official Japanese dietary guidelines are similar to those of the U.S. in that they are high-carbohydrate—which may be surprising to learn, due to the fact that their rates of obesity and related illnesses are dramatically lower than ours. Notably, it is their food preference and eating habits which reduce the incidence of the serious illnesses responsible for draining most of our nation's healthcare budget. To put it simply, the Japanese do not share our culture of overeating. Therefore, we can deduce that we could make great strides to better health simply by adopting this attitude of moderation, even while sticking with our current diet. Switching to the human diet, of course, would push us much further toward our health improvement goals.

Moving us further toward our evolution-aligned nutritional criteria could completely upset the current nutrition-health paradigm—we could discover what the human body is capable of, given the optimal external circumstances. To accomplish this, though, we have to lose our arrogant point of view that, at least in the short term, we can outsmart evolution and arbitrarily establish what and how to eat. The key here is not to confuse thriving with accommodation. After all, we have evolved to prosper in specific dietary conditions, but we have adapted to survive in an even wider set of circumstances. That adaptation resulted in the incredible flexibility of our digestion and is the reason that our bodies tolerate our modern menu. Because of the widening of our geographical roaming range and general accessibility of all types of foods, we have adapted to broad variety in our consumption habits. And thus it's not surprising that we can live eating grains supplemented with meats, dairy, fruit, and vegetables all year round.

We can survive similarly well or even better on any other combination of foods, a fact to which the proponents of the vegetarian, Atkins, Paleo, and other diets can attest. However, that broad accommodation doesn't imply *thriving*. Our bodies can perform at their best only by following the evolution-formed eating model we will explore in subsequent chapters. That model is very different from the popular diets promoted today. Moreover, in some respects, the optimal model goes against many of the entrenched opinions about what is healthy. Unfortunately, while in its outlines the ancestral paradigm is pretty obvious, there is currently not much science behind it. No one appears to be interested in posing the question, "What is the *prototypical human* eating model? The one that is independent of our food production and eating traditions?" The cause of that disinterest is not that surprising, since the bulk of nutritional studies are financed by the food industry. They appear to seek only the convenient confirmation of the health benefits of different takes on the traditional foods and diets. And, unfortunately, studies sponsored by the government explore a similar range of issues. Thus we have a stalemate in pursuing unconventional eating models. Instead of seriously analyzing them, we leave them to the health fanatics and focus on researching more profitable medications. Although it's evident that we have evolved to eat differently than we do now, the experts do not dare to even consider our ancestral nutrition as a valid option.

Part Two

Chapter Two

Imperfect Humans

Have you ever wondered why we are so imperfect? Why do our bodies demand so much maintenance? Other mammals seem to be able to get away with a simple self-care routine. We, on the other hand, have to commit a lot of time and effort to our upkeep. For example, we require extensive oral care to maintain our teeth. Otherwise, we get cavities, plaque, periodontal disease, or halitosis. Many of us have an underdeveloped lower jaw and must bear its consequences, like impacted wisdom teeth. We can correct these issues to a certain degree through orthodontia and oral surgery. But why are we bothered by those problems at all?

And what about our gastrointestinal ailments? To regulate our digestion, we routinely take TUMS, Pepto-Bismol, and various anti-gas, anti-diarrheal, and laxative medications. Why can't our gastrointestinal tract function without discomfort?

Is our skin faring any better? To take care of our dermis, which is either too dry or too oily, we use various creams and lotions. As if that weren't enough, we face many more severe afflictions like rashes, acne, eczema, psoriasis, and rosacea. Adding to our socialization barriers is our not-so-pleasant skin odor. In order to smell agreeable, we need to bathe daily and rely heavily on deodorants.

Autoimmune diseases like seasonal and food allergies plague us, too. Besides lowering our everyday quality of life, they can introduce symptoms like headaches and periods of tiredness or drowsiness. To keep ourselves alert throughout the day, we turn to coffee, tea, and energy drinks. And when at the end of the day we can't fall asleep, we rely on sleeping pills.

Even the occurrence of mental issues is alarmingly high in our society. From ADHD, bulimia, and anorexia to depression and schizophrenia, they seem to be the curse of our modern-day lives. Approximately one in five adults in the U.S.—43.8 million, or 18.5 percent of us—experiences mental illness in a given year. Can we blame all that on the pace of life and the difficulty of "finding ourselves" in the modern world? Or can it be that all these problems are in large part related to our nutrition?

The human body is a complex auto-regulating system constituted of roughly 100 trillion cells. Let that sink in. A hundred, followed by nine zeroes. Our bodies exhibit a level of complexity that is hardly comparable to any machinery we have ever created. They are autonomous universes of cooperating cells that keep us functioning as well as we allow them to. Although it's not immediately apparent to us, we are the host to at least as many microorganisms as there are cells in our body. They include bacteria, fungi, and viruses. They are collectively called human microbiota and their members range from beneficial, to neutral, to hostile. Our bodies continually interact with the microbiota, trying to keep it in balance.

The system that we call the human body is complicated indeed. Adding to the difficulty of studying our bodies are the variations between individuals. We each have a unique genetic makeup responsible for the differences in the ways our cell systems work. That includes our diverse development process and immunity to diseases. Scientists know a lot about our anatomy and the life processes occurring within us. However, due to the astounding level of complexity inherent in these processes, their knowledge is far from complete. While they are familiar with some organs and biochemical systems, others are only fragmentarily understood and still others wholly unexplored. That is why the drug approval process is so lengthy and rigorous. From in vitro experiments to animal and human studies, medications are scrutinized over many years for their safety and efficacy. Even that, as we know, doesn't guarantee that new pharmaceuticals are perfectly safe. There are many cases where, after multiple years on the market, a medication is withdrawn due to its dangerous side effects.

Although our knowledge about some complex systems is limited, it does not, and should not, stop us from making reasonably educated guesses. This is especially true when the actions we take or predictions we make based on such systems are crucial to our well-being. An example of this may be our weather forecasting, where foretelling atmospheric phenomena proves to be very useful despite the lack of absolute certainty. Likewise, medical arts rely on educated guesses to a certain degree, although in most cases, the uncertainty factor is very narrow. Modern medicine has proven itself to be extremely effective. Among countless examples of its competence is the significantly reduced mortality rate achieved through vaccinations, antibiotics, advances in surgery, and recently developed medications for taming HIV.

Both medicine and nutrition operate within the same realm. Both deal with the same complex system—the human body. So why does medicine work so well while nutrition fails so badly? One reason may be that our foods, unlike our drugs, are ruled by a different set of precepts. What we eat profoundly affects our health. The ancients knew that; nobody said it better than Hippocrates in his famous quote, "Let food be thy medicine and medicine be thy food." So why do we treat medicine seriously and nutrition casually? Think about visiting a hospital versus going to a restaurant. They seem to reside on the opposite sides of our life-enjoyment spectrum. Yet they both influence our health. We know that the diet-health link exists, but we bury it somewhere in the back of our minds. Even when feeling sick because of diet, we sooner reach for a supplement or a drug rather than change our way of eating.

We have a hierarchy of health conditions and their equivalent methods of treatment. We use home remedies for the ones that bother us least, then reach for over-the-counter medications for more effectiveness, and when things get serious we turn to doctors for help. We intuitively understand that the more effective the treatment, the more potential for adverse side effects. Hence, between two remedies of similar efficacy, we reach first for the one that we consider less intrusive. That almost benign category is very appealing, and it happens to comprise many natural supplements and foods.

It's pretty common to encounter instances of one of these natural supplements being touted as a wonder remedy for this or that condition. And there are a lot of these benign magic bullets out there. Since the perceived ratio of efficacy to side effects seems high, we are quick to start using them.

Considering ourselves rational thinkers, our general line of reasoning is as follows: "The reason for my *[insert your complaint here]* is that I am missing *[insert miracle cure here]*." By far, the most popular self-administered remedies are vitamins. We reason that since they are necessary, a deficiency of one can throw our body out of balance. Furthermore, if small amounts of certain vitamins are good for us, more of them should be even better. Being very thorough, we research extensively and find the "best" brand. After consuming them for a while, it's hard for us to admit that we see little difference. But then, after a while, we find another miracle cure and repeat the research, hope, disappointment, and abandonment cycle. Doing so, some of us go for years through the long list of "magical" remedies. Here is a short version of that list.

- Minerals
- Antioxidants
- Amino acids
- Prebiotics and probiotics
- Salt water
- Honey
- Water with lemon
- Apple cider vinegar in different concoctions
- Superfoods including quinoa, spirulina, exotic berries, mushrooms, and other "miracle foods of the week" that are being promoted by the media

How much of it is true? The vitamin that most of us lack is vitamin D because it's produced by our bodies when we expose our skin to the sun, which we don't do much nowadays. Another one is vitamin B12, which can be hard to get enough of, on the vegetarian diet in particular.

We consume sufficient amounts of other vitamins while eating mostly random foods.

It's a similar story with minerals. We may be possibly missing some magnesium if our diet is less than perfect; on the other hand, we definitely consume too much sodium.

Amino acids fall into two groups: essential and inessential. As you might guess, we need to ingest the essential ones, and generally, there are enough of them on a regular diet. Our bodies can synthesize inessential amino acids when required.

Antioxidants are substances that contribute to the prevention of cell damage. Various foods and drinks are being advertised as a source of antioxidants. While most of those claims are factually correct, the efficacy of their cell-protective powers is exaggerated. The fact is that we can get enough antioxidants from a varied, healthy diet. Additionally, our bodies can produce their own.

Prebiotics and probiotics keep our bacterial flora in balance. Prebiotic is the fiber needed for the probiotics (bacteria) to live in our gastrointestinal tracts. Supplementing with prebiotics, we try to fix our poor diet by adding the beneficial ingredients that we have already removed from it. With probiotics, we attempt to supply the beneficial bacteria which we killed off by our inappropriate diet.

In a similar vein, we try to fix our health with apple cider vinegar, brine, honey, and other natural substances.

As with our reliance on supplements, we also tend to trust various forms of alternative medicine. We want to believe that megadoses of vitamins can work, as well as spiritual energy, magnets, naturopathy, homeopathy, and so on.

Unfortunately, we are prone to trusting the quackery abounding on the internet. Many of us believe the scholarly-sounding articles on unconventional therapies websites or hang on every word of the guy on YouTube who sounds so very convincingly like he knows what he is talking about.

Focusing on supplements, superfoods, and alternative medicine is seldom a good idea. It's a result of an oversimplified view of our body; an attempt to second-guess the complex auto-regulating system.

We tend to look for simple solutions that we can easily understand, even when they pertain to complex systems. However, sometimes complex solutions are necessary and sometimes tinkering with complicated machinery is just a waste of time.

In many cases, however, trusting alternative healing methods can be outright dangerous. And, even if it isn't, it presents potential harm by distracting us from improving our diet or seeking medical help.

Chapter Three

Cravings

The feelings of taste, craving, and hunger were crucial to our ancestors' survival. They urged them to eat and helped them choose among the available foods. We are genetically the same Stone Age people, shaped by natural selection to survive in the wild. Within a few thousand years, our nutritional environment has completely changed. Is it any surprise that our instincts clash with the modern way of eating?

The same eating impulses that for half a million years helped us survive now contribute to making us overweight and sick. It's important to realize that the factors that encourage or deter us from eating are different than the ones known to our pre-farming ancestors. Here is what changed:

- ❖ Availability of food went from limited to plentiful.
- ❖ Acquiring food went from risky and arduous to safe and easy.
- ❖ Natural fasting associated with food seasonality and scarcity disappeared.
- ❖ Our physical activity decreased.
- ❖ Foods changed from wild/simply-processed to farm-grown/ industrially-processed. As a result, high-calorie foods with super-addictive macronutrient combinations appeared; the content of nutritional fiber decreased.

❖ Salt and other seasonings became commonly available.

❖ The principal purpose of eating shifted from satisfying hunger to an everyday routine or diversion and eating frequency increased as a matter of tradition and easy access.

Many of those factors alone can make us gain weight. Imagine now how the combination of them all affects our food consumption. Except for the decrease in physical activity (which should, in theory, diminish our appetite), all other factors are encouraging us to eat more. Underlying all of them is our primal survival strategy.

Without a doubt, the compulsion to binge on calorie-rich food was essential to our ancestors' survival. It was a way to store extra energy for leaner times. Our bodies can do that by efficiently saving the caloric surplus as body fat. That convenient lipid reserve only depletes when needed for survival. Our species, like other mammals, adapted well to the sporadic nature of food supply, where alternating periods of plentitude and scarcity were not uncommon. What used to be critical to our survival—a practical system of long-term energy buffering— became our modern curse.

Let's look at how the system used to work in practice based on one certain kind of food: the seasonally available wild fruit which helped our forefathers build up a fat store.

Guided by its sweetness, our ancestors, like other animals, most likely ate as much fruit as they could. In other words, they behaved exactly like us in a doughnut shop. For them, however, this appetite for sweetness was a critically important drive. During the period when fruits and other energy-dense foods were in season, our forefathers were able to develop a fat reserve that would help them safely survive through the winter.

Some mammals push that winter survival strategy even further with an ability to hibernate over the coldest, most inhospitable months of the year. Humans can't do that, but building fat reserves for the winter seems perfectly reasonable. The term "scheduled obesity" perfectly describes the true nature of this seasonal overindulgence.

How much fat can one store when adding wild fruit and other carbohydrate-rich foods over a few months? First, let's make some assumptions about seasonal plant foods in those days:

1) They were not as packed with calories as today's cultivated equivalents.

2) Gathering them required considerable effort.

3) Due to their arbitrary nutrient density, they required preparation to make them sufficiently nutritious. Thus, the most nourishing parts were most likely extracted, broken up, and possibly cooked.

The harvesting and preparation of plant food from wild sources, even with a relatively bountiful foraging area, couldn't have supplied too many calories. Thus, our ancestors certainly could gain some weight, but not enough to make them overweight by today's standard. Modern-defined "obesity" would endanger Paleo humans' survival by significantly impairing their mobility.

The sensitivity of our senses of taste and smell is a crucial factor in our food choices. As much as our ancestors could appreciate the richness of food, they knew only the taste of simply processed plants, fish, and game meats. Obviously, they didn't have access to the elaborate taste-enhancing techniques we use today. And, as their taste wasn't blunted by the use of seasonings and processed foods, they were more sensitive to the nutritional and toxic properties of their meals.

Even though we have radically modified our foods and the ways we consume them, we can't escape being controlled by the same precivilizational eating impulses, which make us favor and binge on calorie-loaded dishes. To make matters worse, we excel in improving the taste of our food. A more enjoyable eating experience drives us to consume more.

As individuals, we can each control our cravings to a different extent —and only very few of us can sufficiently rein in our eating drives. Most of us are incapable of resisting the allure of calories. Although we use the term "addiction" in reference to the most extreme cases, all of us feel an instinctive, powerful craving for high-calorie dishes. For example, it's difficult to refuse a burger with fries and a sweet drink. To our brains, a meal like that presents a highly desirable macronutrient mother lode. After all, it consists of highly concentrated proteins, fats, and loads of carbohydrates. Of the three, carbs are what we crave most. To our survival-geared brains, the taste of sugary and starchy foods is a promise of an almost instant energy supply. As we consume the rewarding food, we form memories of the satisfying taste and the alluring smell associated with its richness. And, after frequent reinforcement, whenever we smell, see, or imagine the delicious carb-y treats, we crave them. However, we should realize that those enticing refined carbs shouldn't be our everyday nourishment; our bodies are not attuned to consuming them on a regular basis in large quantities. How do we know that? Through the frequent occurrences of diet-related ailments, which vary from common indigestion to type 2 diabetes and cancers. Even our dental issues can indicate that there is a problem with the bacterial flora thriving on concentrated starches in our mouths. After all, without frequent brushing and cleaning, the bacteria feeding on the carbs between our teeth cause a whole range of dental problems, ranging from cavities and plaque to periodontal disease. Even with daily brushing and flossing, most of us need to visit the dentist for periodic teeth cleaning due to bacterial plaque buildup. How does the addictive nature of refined carbs manifest in real life?

First, through smell. Carb-y foods smell so good because they evoke pleasant taste memories. That's why it's hard to pass by a bakery without noticing the smell of freshly baked goodies. One experiences a similar sensation when inhaling the aroma of french fries.

The sense of smell is a strong encourager to commit to that first bite.

Once the taste combined with the smell starts working on our brain, we can't stop eating. A good illustration of this phenomenon may be the line from that old Lay's potato chip commercial: "Bet you can't eat just one!" And that, unlike the claims in most commercials, is very true. We typically keep reaching for the carb-y snack until it's gone. Finishing a portion of a carb-y meal is not the end of its influence on our brain. The idea about the availability of the carbohydrates remains in our subconsciousness. And, when after an hour or two our insulin level goes back down, guess what emerges? Yes, the craving to eat more carbs. That is the time when we reach for the leftovers of our meal. Just one portion of carbs can create a longer-term subconscious want. That increased awareness of carbohydrates doesn't stop when we cease to eat them. Even when we lower their content in our meals, it usually lasts about two weeks. And during that period, starchy or sugary foods seem especially tempting. While in that carb-sensitive mode, we have to exercise a lot of willpower to resist the temptation to indulge.

People starting on low-carb diets report that only after several weeks of dieting do they no longer feel the same level of craving for carbohydrate-rich foods.

It is fascinating to me why this strong attraction to carbs wanes after a few weeks. It is as though, after the period of being compelled to overeat, we are given another chance to evaluate our foods with a clear head.

And here, once more, we bump into the curse of the steady food supply. Unlike our pre-farming ancestors who only had sporadic access to carb-y foods, we have a constant supply of them. And thus, most of us get stuck in the high starch-craving mode.

Chapter Four

Reasons for Overeating

The way we nourish our bodies is unquestionably crucial to our health. And, although we are told otherwise, the responsibility for our poor nutrition is not entirely ours. We don't live in a bubble, and thus our choice of foods is based on many external factors.

First and foremost are **availability, price, and marketing**. Many businesses compete to offer us economical meals, including big fast food corporations looking to satisfy our appetites on the go. These companies are widely present, with a huge number of locations across the country. To illustrate my point, here is the list of the most popular fast food places with their corresponding number of locations in the world.

---

[2] "List of the largest fast food restaurant chains." *Wikipedia.* Accessed October 3, 2018. **https://en.wikipedia.org/wiki/List_of_the_largest_ fast_food_restaurant_chains.**

Company	Number of Locations
Subway	43,015
McDonald's	37,200
Starbucks	28,720
KFC	20,404
Burger King	16,859
Pizza Hut	16,796
Domino's Pizza	15,000
Dunkin' Donuts	11,300
Baskin-Robbins	7,500
Hunt Brothers Pizza	7,300
Taco Bell	7,000
Wendy's	6,490

What kind of foods are most prominently featured and offered as the best deals on the menu? Here is a sample promotion from one of the big fast food chains:

- ¼-lb. Cheeseburger for $1
- FREE FRIES WITH PURCHASE OF $1+
- GET A BREAKFAST SANDWICH FOR $2
- Fries, ¼-lb. Cheeseburger and Hamburger GET $2 OFF a $10+ purchase

The offers are, in fact, exceptional deals considering the calories contained in the meals. That fact, combined with the widespread accessibility, fast service, and powerful advertising, makes fast food places our favorites.

The second food choice factor is **its energy density and consequently its level of enticement.** We are naturally attracted to caloric meals, especially those containing a high carbohydrate/fat combination. That is the reason we prefer fries, pizzas, doughnuts, burgers, hot dogs, and sandwiches accompanied by sweet drinks instead of salads washed down with water. Our attraction to the high-caloric combos is, in many cases, making our food choices for us. Although rarely mentioned in the context of everyday food consumption, the addictiveness of our modern foods is a real problem. Memories of the tasty carbs, fats, and sugars in various combinations compel us to go back over and over to our same "favorite" foods.

The third factor affecting our food choice is **social pressure**. Unfortunately, we feel a significant cultural pressure to eat super-caloric food. That, combined with our natural attraction to it and its addictive nature, makes adhering to a lower-calorie diet very tough. For example, imagine refusing a piece of cake at a birthday party or a family function. Pretty much all shared meals exert some pressure to participate. In the same vein, unless the whole family commits to healthy eating, separate meal preparation for one person becomes very cumbersome.

The fourth factor is **misinformation**. That includes both inadequate and wrong information. Guided by the official recommendations, most of us consider our random high-carbohydrate diets appropriate for everyday consumption. And, in fact, concerning the macronutrient ratio, most Americans comply with government-backed nutritional guidelines. From that point of view, pizza, pasta, sandwiches, and burgers are all wholly recommended. Although there is nothing inherently wrong with those foods, consuming them as a part of the three-meals-a-day routine can undoubtedly lead to overeating. Additionally, the majority of Americans adhere to the recommendation to restrict their fat consumption. In doing so, they consume just enough fat with the starches to make the combination super-addictive. Another example is the prominent recommendation of fruits. Sugar is addictive and, even in the guise of fruit, should be consumed in moderation. It looks like we are advised to frequently eat a variety of highly addictive foods—and the fault for the overindulgence is entirely laid upon us.

In general, the government's dietary guide reads like a food industry sales brochure. While imposing limits on highly processed foods, it simultaneously promotes them merely by inclusion among viable menu choices. The problem is that those foods are usually also habit-forming; therefore, advice like that is akin to recommending a smoker indulge in just a few puffs of a cigarette. Furthermore, the nutrient labels on foods available in our markets are pretty useless. They list macronutrient content in grams per arbitrarily established servings, which makes it hard to make a correct intake estimation. Not many Americans can visualize the weight of consumed food, especially in grams. The volume indicated in teaspoons, tablespoons, or cups and percentages would make more sense. Also, the food labels don't show how a given food compares to others regarding macronutrient ratio or fiber content.

The fifth factor affecting our food choices is **a little more subtle**. Due to the popularity of calorie-loaded meals, we tend to thoughtlessly accept them as wholesome nourishment. Pretty much any home-cooked dish *seems* to be healthy. In other words, while being aware of fast food restaurants as providers of junk food, most of us consider home-cooked equivalents as better. Thus, a home-baked pizza, chicken pot pie, or eggs with bacon, buttered toast, and orange juice fall into the category of approved sustenance. And for those who can stick to strict portion control, these foods are okay. However, they invite binging and, as part of the three-meals-daily plan, can easily push us over the daily calorie limit.

Based on the above food selection influencers, one can see how difficult it is not to overeat and what an effort it is to stay on a restrictive diet surrounded by the myriad of temptations. As is typical with addictions, we surrender to the enticement when there is immediate availability. That makes just driving by burger places or doughnut shops a trying experience. We experience the same reaction walking down the supermarket aisles, where we are assaulted by the smells and sights of sweet, fatty, and starchy delights.

Chapter Five

Nutritional Guides

Shaping the food supply starts with food production. The most profitable agricultural products which are also the easiest to process are clear winners for the food industry—especially if at the same time, they keep the customer coming back for more.

The government recommends limiting consumption of certain foods while it also, through subsidies, makes those same foods cheaper to the consumer. For example, the infamous high fructose corn syrup commonly used in processed foods is made from government-subsidized corn. Similarly supported is wheat, which, once converted into white flour, is one of the main culprits of the obesity epidemic. Overall, the de facto regulation of the agriculture industry through subsidies pushes the food market in an unhealthy direction.

The other prong of the government's influence on the public's food consumption takes the form of dietary recommendations. The scientists responsible for establishing official guidelines are guilty of, at the very least, equivocation: They consider all foods available on the market as worthy of recommendation. Let's examine the advice from the aforementioned 2015-2020 Dietary Guidelines. Item number three reads, "Limit calories from added sugars and saturated fats and reduce sodium intake." That seems an underhanded recommendation to keep consuming added sugars. Also, while warning about saturated fats, on whose unhealthy nature the jury is still out, the authors of this advice don't mention the possibly more dangerous trans fats. Also—what form of sodium should we avoid? Why there is no specific mention of salt? Should we check our vegetables for sodium content? Or merely stop adding salt to our foods?

The guidelines recommend grains and fruit as a part of the healthy eating pattern in the following bullet points: "Fruits, especially whole fruits"; grains, at least half of which are whole grains." Here again, processed grains and candied and dried fruit are allowed on the menu. Why are these highly questionable foods recommended at all? Why are the authors of these guidelines so politically correct as to include pretty much *all* foods in their recommendations?

The word "limit," when pertaining to sugar and salt, should be replaced with the word "avoid" in order to send an appropriately strong message. What calamity would cause the exclusion of extra sugar and overprocessed foods from our diet? Apart from reducing diabetes and cancer rates, this change would put quite a few dentists out of business.

Overall, the Guidelines' approach is flawed. Rather than correcting our distorted line of thinking about food, it follows it. We have to realize that even though we have grown accustomed to them, the bulk of the currently available foods are not the ones we evolved to consume. The truth is that we created them without regard for our health. We wanted to feed more people with fewer crops. And thus our staples developed into incredibly dense calorie sources.

It took a long time to get our crops to their current forms. The modern, heavily processed foods are just the latest stage of the continual "improvement" process started ten thousand years ago by our first farmers. But being stuck with modern foods doesn't mean that we can't imitate the real hunter-gatherer diet.

The Paleolithic (or "Paleo") diet recommends the following macronutrient ratios (as a percentage of calories):

- Fat: 27-47%
- Carbohydrate: 22-40%
- Protein: 19-35%

In contrast, the government's recommended Accepted Macronutrient Distribution Ranges (AMDR) for adults (as a percentage of calories) are as follows:

- Fat: 20-35%
- Carbohydrate: 45-65%
- Protein: 10-35%

Below are two tables showing how some popular meals compare to the AMDR and Paleo diet recommendations. The numbers preceded with signs indicate how far the meal varies from the recommended limit. For example, -2 indicates 2% below the lower limit, while +3 shows 3% above the upper limit. The column marked FR (fiber ratio) shows the fiber content expressed as the ratio of fiber (in grams) to total calories, normalized for 1,000 calories. The computation of the ratio is as follows: FR = [fibers in grams] x 1,000/[total calories].

For example, let's compute the fiber ratio of a Big Mac meal with a large fry and a large Coke, which has 9 grams of total fiber and 1,340 total calories. Thus FR = (9 x 1,000)/1,340 = 6.7. The USDA recommends 14 grams of fiber per 1,000 calories.[3]

---

[3] U.S. Department of Agriculture. **"The Food Supply and Dietary Fiber: Its Availability and Effect on Health. Nutrition Insight 36."** Accessed October 3, 2018. **https://www.cnpp.usda.gov/sites/default/files/ nutrition_insights_uploads/Insight36.pdf.**

CARBOHYDRATE-BASED MEALS

Food	Fat	Carbs	Protein	Fiber Ratio
Pepperoni Pizza (549 cal., 4.8g fiber)	34.3	43	19	8.7
AMDR Diet Difference		-2		
Paleo Diet Difference		+3		
Burger, Fries, Soda (1,340 cal., 9g fiber)	34.9	53.7	9.5	6.7
AMDR Diet Difference			-0.5	
Paleo Diet Difference		+13.7	-9.5	
Fettuccine Alfredo (1,010 cal., 7g fiber)	49.9	36.5	11.9	6.9
AMDR Diet Difference	+14.9	-9.4		
Paleo Diet Difference	+2.9		-7.1	

SALADS

Food	Fat	Carbs	Protein	Fiber Ratio
Buffalo Chicken (970 cal., 4g fiber)	61.2	16.4	20.2	4.1
AMDR Diet Difference		-28.6		
Paleo Diet Difference		-5.6		
Grilled Chicken (700 cal., 8g fiber)	33.4	44	30.2	11.4
AMDR Diet Difference		-1		
Paleo Diet Difference		+4		
Santa Fe Chicken (940 cal., 10g fiber)	66	17	14	10.6
AMDR Diet Difference	+31	-28		
Paleo Diet Difference	+19	-5	-5	
Cobb (370 cal., 5g fiber)	56	15.1	25.9	13.5
AMDR Diet Difference	+21	-29.9		
Paleo Diet Difference	+9	-6.1		

The upper table shows that the macronutrient ratio is closer to the AMDR recommendations. The lower table shows that the macronutrient ratio is—except for the Grilled Chicken Salad—closer to the Paleo recommendations. Therefore, most of the salads are within the Paleo macronutrient ranges. On the other hand, the typical fast food combos fit in the high-carbohydrate diet (AMDR) nutritional brackets.

Note that none of the meals listed in the tables reach the recommended fiber ratio of 14 grams per thousand calories. Also, except for the McDonald's meal, none contain drinks. Adding a caloric drink further reduces the fiber ratio; for example, the Big Mac meal with a large fry and Diet Coke (or water) has the FR of 8.6. For the same combo with Diet Coke replaced by regular Coke, the FR drops to 6.7.

Dietary fiber is essential to our health. It is like a catalyst required for the proper functioning of our digestive system. Here is a relevant abstract published by the National Institutes of Health:[4]

Dietary fiber intake provides many health benefits. However, average fiber intakes for U.S. children and adults are less than half of the recommended levels. Individuals with high intakes of dietary fiber appear to be at significantly lower risk for developing coronary heart disease, stroke, hypertension, diabetes, obesity, and certain gastrointestinal diseases. Increasing fiber intake lowers blood pressure and serum cholesterol levels. Increased intake of soluble fiber

---

[4] National Center for Biotechnology Information (NCBI). **"Health benefits of dietary fiber."** Accessed October 3, 2018. **https://www.ncbi.nlm.nih.gov/pubmed/19335713**.

improves glycemia and insulin sensitivity in non-diabetic and diabetic individuals. Fiber supplementation in obese individuals significantly enhances weight loss. Increased fiber intake benefits some gastrointestinal disorders including the following: gastroesophageal reflux disease, duodenal ulcer, diverticulitis, constipation, and hemorrhoids. Prebiotic fibers appear to enhance immune function. Dietary fiber intake provides similar benefits for children as for adults.

To get some idea about the fiber and carbohydrate content of different foods, let's compare a few of them, keeping in mind that the recommended fiber density is 14 grams per thousand kilocalories (kCal).

Fiber Density per 1,000 kCal

Food	Fiber Density
Ham Sandwich	2.6
Milk Chocolate Bar	4.5
Cookies	6.3
Sweet Cereal	6.5
White Bread	10.1
Spaghetti	11.3
French Fries	12
Corn Flakes Cereal	12.5
Watermelon	12.9
RECOMMENDED DENSITY	14
Whole Bread	27.5
Banana	29.5
Apple	46.3
Strawberry	50
Tomato	66.7
Broccoli	76
Bell Pepper	83.3
Lettuce, Green Leaf	100
Avocado	427

While the recommended fiber intake is 14 grams per thousand calories, the nutritional labels don't list the fiber density as shown in the table. An even more illustrative version of the fiber content relative to its recommended value would be the deviation from the recommended density. That parameter could be presented as: [fiber density] - 14 = [fiber saturation index].

The modified table would look as follows:

Fiber Saturation Index (FSI)

Food	FSI
Ham Sandwich	-11.4
Milk Chocolate Bar	-9.5
Cookies	-7.7
Sweet Cereal	-7.5
White Bread	-3.9
Spaghetti	-27
French Fries	-2
Corn Flakes Cereal	-1.5
Watermelon	-1.1
RECOMMENDED DENSITY	0
Whole Bread	13.5
Banana	15.5
Apple	32.3
Strawberry	36
Tomato	52.7
Broccoli	62
Bell Pepper	69.3
Lettuce, Green Leaf	86
Avocado	413

Having a straightforward fiber content indicator like the FSI on nutritional labels would be useful for consumers. The sign of the index shows whether adding the food adds or reduces fiber relative to the consumption goal of 14g/1,000kCal. The value indicates the deviation from the recommended amount.

Chapter Six

Obsession

You may find what I am about to say in this chapter a little controversial. It's because many of us have an emotional connection to food. However, I feel strongly that our infatuation with sustenance is a significant factor contributing to our nutritional predicament.

Our ancestors ate to survive, whereas we mostly treat our nourishment as a mood enhancer. Anytime we need an emotional uplift, it's time for another meal or an occasion for a snack. Those "food breaks" are an excellent diversion from daily routine and a mini-celebration. From the decision on what to eat, through the shopping or cooking, up to that last gratifying bite, it's all pleasure. Although some of us don't like cooking at home, we all love to sit down to an already prepared meal. That is why we enjoy dining out so much. Either accompanied or solo, meals seem to taste better in the welcoming surrounding of a restaurant. The novelty of different establishments and a variety of dishes often make culinary outings a regular activity for us.

Being social animals, the company of others makes our eating experience much more gratifying. We like to dine with our dates, family, and business acquaintances.

As with adding a companion to our dining experience, we also like to combine eating with entertainment; as pleasurable a diversion as it may be by itself, combining it with munching significantly intensifies the pleasure. To fully realize that distinct eating opportunity, we invented specialized snack foods. Having that helpful nourishment, we can do something entertaining while casually grazing on potato chips, pretzels, or popcorn. In case we forget about that activity intensification system, we can always rely on ubiquitous and vigorous snack food advertising.

The term "comfort food" exemplifies another notorious eating attitude. Often when faced with difficulties, we cheer ourselves up with a filling, satisfying meal. In short, we can't complain about the shortage of occasions, pretexts, and excuses to eat.

The central focus of our food culture is cooking. Nutritionists recommend it as a means to encourage healthy eating. Most of us agree and consider it a valuable skill. After all, cooking a nutritious meal at home may be the best way to avoid the temptations of reaching for the ubiquitous fast food.

We view the kitchen as the most important room in the house. We find that special room to be charming due to its inviting utilitarian nature and its role as a family hub. After all, it's where we bond as families and socialize with friends.

Everything related to food preparation and consumption is highly valued in our culture, and the cooking-enthusiastic attitude is considered positive and worth promoting. And, when contrasted with eating random junk foods, it certainly is. However, the cooking affection became more than encouragement to eat healthily—it became a societal obsession. That obsession pushes the nutritional aspect of cooking to the background. In our view, meals have become a way to express our creativity. We look for ways to make them always fresh and original. In that pursuit, we feel the need to make them look, smell, and taste the best they can be. That striving for fulfillment through cooking shows up in our over-the-top appreciation of celebrity chefs, cooking TV shows, and best-selling cookbooks. We not only *like* to cook and eat; many of us are *fascinated* by nearly every aspect of food preparation and consumption. We create an aura of festivity around our sustenance. That attitude is profoundly rooted in our culture, as our celebrations are centered around sumptuous meals. We are so caught up in the culinary lifestyle that we don't realize the extent of its artifice.

The plain fact is that we overemphasize the significance of our nourishment and its preparation. Modern cooking looks very different when assessed unemotionally. In fact, it is just another form of processing whose chief purpose is to enhance food's taste. When all the glamour is stripped from the act, we can see elaborate cooking for what it really is: a way to intensify our food cravings.

I remember being annoyed with my mother for calling me for meals as a kid. I considered it an unnecessary disruption of my daily activities. Eating on a schedule was a chore. I felt that I shouldn't be compelled to eat when not hungry. I liked playing on an empty stomach, and usually, I didn't even realize when I was hungry. It just felt normal. But the societal pressure to join in for family meals won out. Eventually, in my late teenage years, I got used to clock-imposed meals, thereby suppressing my natural instincts. And then I started feeling odd and uneasy without any food in my belly. Thoughts of and plans for my next meal inserted themselves into my everyday thinking routine.

Scheduled eating is in no way natural. It's something that we are trained in from early childhood. The result of this habit is a feeling of uneasiness when our stomachs are empty. We are so used to constant digestion that we consider the normal empty-stomach state as something highly unusual and therefore uncomfortable; we learn to misinterpret it as hunger.

We have to make the distinction between two kinds of communal eating—frequent and on-schedule, or sufficiently planned for when the participants are actually hungry. Combining eating with socializing is not a modern invention; it had been a way of life for our nomadic predecessors. However, there was an important difference between our business dinners and our ancestors' communal meals. Notably, we sit at our dinner table after consuming two prior meals that day, while they did so on empty stomachs.

Despite that difference, during our scheduled dining, we mutually exert on ourselves the pressure to eat. We are so used to collective eating that we feel uncomfortable when a person at the table declines to participate.

It's understandable that mealtimes are a matter of practicality when food is prepared at home. However, scheduled, frequent eating goes against our natural pattern.

It's interesting to consider why we want our meals to be extra-appetizing. Our level of craving for food is a combination of two factors: our level of hunger and the taste of the meal. Exceptional flavor and aroma motivate us to eat when we are not hungry. And thus we prepare delicious meals to stay on the feeding schedule. Toward that end, we use copious amounts of food seasoning. Without a second thought, we use salt, pepper, salad dressings, shredded cheese, and myriad other taste enhancers. In other words, we go out of our way to make ourselves overeat.

Chapter Seven

Addiction

Let's revisit a very controversial subject related to obesity: food addiction. This topic is highly disputed. Many nutritionists insist that food, being a necessity for survival, cannot be considered addictive. They say that even though eating patterns like abstention and binging resemble addictive patterns, certain foods can be considered highly palatable, but not at the level of "addictive." The fact that those highly palatable, often super-caloric foods are forbidden is the cause of our vicious restrictions/overeating patterns.

The above exemplifies a typical quibbling on the subject. I beg to disagree with the benign characterization of the foods that create the dependency; I think that harmful eating patterns are the result of the addictive nature of the foods in question. Not only are those calorie-packed foods addictive, but the fact that they are is not surprising at all—it's the result of our evolutionary adaptation. The foods, their common consumption patterns, and their availability used to be completely different when humans were hunter-gatherers. Hence, the abnormal attraction to certain foods (or ingredients in our foods) which we experience used to contribute to our very survival. The highly caloric foods that we've invented are much more refined compared to the ones available to pre-farming humans. And, therefore, even though they are still considered foods, they are in fact powerfully addictive.

Of course, the levels to which we crave those foods vary depending on the individual, but the inherent powerful instinct to crave and overeat is there in all of us. The reason we lack instinctive "brakes" when consuming carbohydrates, fats, and salt is that in nature we rarely encountered those things in high concentration. And whenever we did, we were justifiably compelled to overindulge. That strong compulsion to binge when food was of higher nutritional quality ensured our survival in times of scarcity. Thus, for our forefathers, the tendency to overeat meant better chances of survival.

If we are genetically programmed to overeat on calorie-rich, simply-processed foods, how much stronger is the drive when it comes to foods that are almost pure carbohydrates and fats or a combination of both? What is surprising about the food addiction issue is that it seems to be not of much interest to the scientific community. We have a myriad of studies surrounding rare eating disorders, and yet we neglect to address the central aspect of the obesity epidemic. On the other hand, maybe we don't need such a study. Perhaps our reality—our society full of millions of overweight people—is the ultimate study in food addiction. Barring more drastic measures, we should at least point out potentially addictive foods. Why don't we implement a simple guide on our food labels to this end?

For example, we could place a color-coded indicator of potential food cravings. That value could be the percentage of net carbohydrates by weight. We could call it "net carbohydrate content" (NCC) and highlight it with different colors depending on the possible addictiveness of the food. Safe foods with low carbohydrate content (less than 5%) could be shown in green, moderately addictive (between 5% and 15%) in yellow, and highly addictive (above 15%) in red.

Let's take a look at how foods fare when classified by their carbohydrate content.

Net Carbohydrate Content (NCC)

Food	NCC
LOW (green)	
Lettuce, Green Leaf	1.39
Avocado	1.4
Tomato	3.3
Bell Pepper	3.36
Broccoli	4.2
MODERATE (yellow)	
Watermelon	6.9
Strawberry	7.5
Apple	13.7
HIGH (red)	
Ham Sandwich	19
Banana	21.9
Spaghetti	28.9
Whole Bread	39.6
French Fries	41
White Bread	47.3
Milk Chocolate Bar	55.8
Cookies	70.6
Corn Flakes Cereal	80.8
High-Sugar Cereal	82.6

The official nutritional guides highly encourage a variety of foods in a diet. One would think that it's one of the most critical aspects of healthy nutrition. Is it indeed? How varied was the menu of our Paleolithic predecessors? It surely fluctuated with the seasons and their current foraging area. The critical difference is that our Paleolithic diet included significant variations in macronutrient ratios, while the modern diet variation is based on the diversity of foods. Thus, the current menu varies foods while keeping the high-carbohydrate profile of our meals. Can the food diversity available to the Paleolithic human be compared to the variety of foods available in our supermarkets? Not by a long shot.

Let's look at the issue from another perspective. Do we need sugar, cookies, chocolate, sweet fruit, dairy, refined grain products, or various overprocessed foods in our diet to stay healthy? No; we can manage just fine without them. In fact, adding them to the menu is risky. Especially consumed in super-addictive combinations, they are powerfully attractive, and many of them provide little to no vitamins, minerals, or fiber. One can argue that fruit and dairy provide some fiber, vitamins, and minerals and thus deserve a recommendation. It's true that they may occasionally be consumed, especially when combined with other foods. However, why should we recommend them if we have healthier alternatives? It seems that the guides include those foods as a way of preserving our long-standing eating tradition and perhaps their associated food industry. And that would be fine, as long as we were informed of the reason. As it is, many of us may assume that a cheese sandwich, orange juice, and milk and cookies are integral parts of the recommended diet variation and that skipping these robs us of important nutrients.

It's difficult to deal with dietary issues because of our wide omnivorous range. Since our bodies are very adaptable biological machines, we can live for a while on pretty much any food that is not too toxic. Determining what's best is the subject of long-standing debates which have resulted in a proliferation of eating recommendations. Among others, we have high-carb, low-carb, keto, Paleo, vegetarian, Mediterranean, and Atkins diets. All of them tout their merits, relying on accompanying studies which seem to back their claims. Most of them focus on specific macronutrient ratios. Maybe they are all right, at least to a degree. Perhaps our bodies can extract what they need from almost any macronutrient mix and adjust themselves accordingly. Possibly the reason that we do better on one diet over another is based on our hereditary predisposition. After all, we have been living in different areas of the globe for millennia, eating different locally available foods. The breadth of our eating adaptation doesn't mean that all foods are equally suitable for us; some of them we tolerate better than others in the long term.

Like other apes, we started as vegetarians, eating raw plant food. Then we adapted to supplement our menu with small amounts of meat. A major change in our eating adaptation which moved us ahead of other animals in terms of foraging range was our ability to process our food. That change, stemming from early humans' ingenuity, allowed us to extract much more nutrition from the surrounding plants and game. Relatively recent is our accommodation of dairy. However, diet is more than particular foods: It's the combination and the frequency of consumption of each. In that sense, we didn't have enough time to adjust to the modern diet. Therefore, our industrially-farmed and super-processed plants and meats consumed throughout all waking hours are something we can tolerate but cannot thrive off of.

While most diets focus on *what* we eat, perhaps as important is *how* we eat. The transition to farming meant not only a change of foods but also a change to the frequency of meals. As a consequence of having a steady supply of starchy foods, we started to eat regularly throughout the day to keep fueling our bodies with quickly-assimilating starch. Having an almost constant food supply meant that fasting became an anomaly rather than a common pattern.

Since then, our menu remains grain-based, augmented with dairy and meat. They are the source of most macronutrients in our diet. Grains are rich in carbohydrates, the dairy and meats in fats and protein. All three are very solid nutritional sources. Out of them, especially starches combined with fats form an irresistible blend. There is a reason for that tasty synergy. Starches are the quickest to make it into the bloodstream, and fats are the densest energy carriers. They seem to complement each other. The fats significantly enhance the taste of carbohydrates—think fries, doughnuts, ice cream, peanut butter with jelly, and bread with butter.

Let's ponder that for a moment. The foods containing one concentrated macronutrient, while tolerable, are not as attractive as the combination of them. The combinations make the food much more crave-able! Like sugar, the aggregate of refined macronutrients and seasonings compels us to overeat. Let's consider the following addictive foods.

French fries = potato + oil + salt = (carbs) + (fat) + (sodium)
Doughnuts = dough + oil + sugar = (carbs) + (fat) + (sugar)
Burger = bun + meat patty = (carbs) + (protein + fat)
Cereal and milk = (carbs + sugar) + (fat + protein + lactose (sugar))
Peanut butter and jelly = (carbs + fat + protein) + (sugar)

Typical in those examples is the combination of concentrated carbohydrates and fats. Adding fat to the carb-y food makes it much more tempting. Note how much of the carbohydrate-rich food we consume with added fat.

That is the reason deep-fried foods are so popular. Deep frying involves covering the food to be fried with batter (a starchy paste) and fusing it with fat. Similarly, adding cheese increases the addictive factor of any starchy food (bread, pasta, pizza, and so forth).

Let's look at how the taste of foods changes when adding different macronutrients. Think of the flavor of refined starches like potatoes or bread on their own. They don't seem very appealing. After adding a fat like butter, however, the flavor improves significantly. Salt or some other seasoning boosts the taste even further.

The mix of the flavors of calorie-dense foods is much more addictive than one would expect by simply evaluating the ingredients separately. In other words, the resulting addictive force is much stronger than the sum of its components; it's more like the product of their original flavors. It's unsurprising that the combination of concentrated desirable substances invokes intense craving. As modern humans, we've gotten accustomed to that reaction in our brain. However, that level of craving was exceptional to our Stone Age ancestors. The flavor of unsalted lean meat or fibrous, starchy, or slightly sweet plant food provided a subdued intensity in their mouths; on the other hand, the taste of a doughnut, French fries, pizza, milkshake, ice cream, or chocolate resides on a different planet in the human culinary universe. As we are still biologically Stone Age people, evolution has not prepared us for that level of temptation.

Part Three

Chapter Eight

In Search of the Human Diet

Let's take a look at our modern diet.

According to the Standard American Diet (SAD)[5], here are the amounts of calories per day that we get from various foods:

Grain Products: 581

Added Plant-Based Fats and Oils: 518

Meat, Poultry, and Fish: 416

Caloric Sweeteners: 369

Dairy: 234

Fruits and Vegetables: 227

How does our current diet compare to our ancestral menu?

From what we know, our forefathers ate mostly meat

---

[5] U.S. Department of Agriculture Economic Research Service. **"A Look at Calorie Sources in the American Diet"** From Chart: "Seventy percent of Americans' calories in 2010 were from plant-based foods" Accessed October 3, 2018. **https:// www.ers.usda.gov/amber-waves/2016/december/a-look-at-calorie-sources-in-the-american-diet/**

and fish augmented with varied plant-sourced food containing a moderate amount of fiber. Therefore, grain products which rank highest on the modern menu were near the bottom of the list for the hunter-gatherers. There were virtually no significant contributors to their diets in the dairy and caloric sweetener categories; the fats composition was also considerably different in those times, as our ancestors did not add refined fats to their meals. However, our forefathers could have supplemented their menu seasonally with nuts, seeds, and other oily plants. The game meat they hunted varied in fat content with the season. Thus, their diet had a higher content of animal fat in the colder months, which suggests that before the year-round availability of fattened, farm-raised meat and dairy, the proportions of animal fats to plant-sourced foods in our diet used to vary with the season. Therefore, the steady addition of animal fat to high quantities of starch is a farm-era consumption model. And, as mentioned before, it's a highly addictive one. Wild fruit, also available seasonally, was most likely not as sugar-packed as today's varieties. However, it was unquestionably very desirable due to its exceptional sweetness.

When considering edible plant foods in our current food assortment, eating fruit every day is highly problematic. As discussed, fruit used to be a contributor to seasonal programmed obesity for the hunter-gatherer. However, for us, it's available all year round and it is a pleasure more than a necessity. Like our ancestors, we crave it for its sweetness. Unlike them, however, we can't complain about the lack of carbohydrates in our diet. Modern fruit does not have a comparable amount of vitamins, minerals, and fiber to vegetables, and it contains plenty of sugar.

The predominant type of sugar contained in fruit is fructose.

Fructose is more suitable to be converted to and deposited as fat rather than used up as a direct energy source. Thus, wild fruit was perfect for our forefathers to build their wintery body fat reserve.

Out of the myriad of dieting recommendations, which one makes the most sense? Should we rely on the official dietary guides and studies? And if so, which of the different recommendations should we follow? In the U.S., the official nutritional guide is far from universally accepted.

For example, Harvard School of Public Health has its own variation of the My Plate brochure, with different emphasis on various foods. Other countries have their separate recommendations. Notably, in many of them, the fruit group loses its prominence. The Canadian guide, for example, reverses the word order in the "Fruit and Vegetable" group to "Vegetable and Fruit." The Japanese guide deprecates fruit even further by making it a separate group located at the end of the list. As varied in details as the national guides are, they all make starchy food staples and promote them as the chief source of calories. Thus, high-carbohydrate consumption advice seems to be a global phenomenon.

We have no reference point showing us how well we could perform eating like true hunter-gatherers while enjoying the advantages of our civilizational progress. However, we can compare the pre-farming diet with the modern diet structure.

Let's take a look. On the one hand, anthropologists show us a rough composition of early humans' diet. On the other, the U.S. government tells us what our macronutrient ratio should be.

	Carbohydrates	Proteins	Fats	Dietary fiber per day
(Early) Humans[6]	22-40%	19-35%	28-58%	45-100g
Recommended (AMDR)[7]	45-65%	10-35%	20-35%	28g
Actual (SAD)[8]	50%	15%	35%	15g

As the difference between macronutrient contributions is quite significant, let's consider the following questions: Why does the current recommendation differ so significantly from the early human diet? And why was that particular nutrient ratio chosen?

We know we can live for a while on a wide range of different foods. However, what makes one macronutrient ratio better than the other? What should be the criteria for the choice? For example, there are scientific studies that show the advantages of the low-carbohydrate diet over the traditional high-carbohydrate diet for weight loss. They also confirm that neither causes significant adverse health effects.

---

[6] Cordain, L., S.B. Eaton, J.B. Miller, and K. Hill. **"The paradoxical nature of hunter-gatherer diets: meat-based, yet non-atherogenic."** *PubMed.* Eur J Clin Nutr., March 2002, 56 Suppl1:S42-52. Accessed October 3, 2018. **https://www.ncbi.nlm.nih.gov/pubmed/11965522.**

[7] Manore, M.M. **"Exercise and the Institute of Medicine recommendations for nutrition."** *PubMed.* Curr Sports Med Rep., August 4, 2005 (4):193-8. Accessed October 3, 2018. **https://www.ncbi.nlm.nih.gov/pubmed/16004827.**

[8] **"Western pattern diet."** *Wikipedia.* Accessed October 3, 2018. **https://en.wikipedia.org/wiki/Western_pattern_diet.**

So why the official recommendation regarding starches?

Curiously, the promoted high-carbohydrate diet is in line with our centuries-old grain-focused farming. Is it a happy coincidence that our nutritional needs correspond to the efficiency-dictated choice of the staple crop? It's as if the farming pioneers, without extensive double-blind studies, had the wise foresight of selecting the healthiest food for mass cultivation. They introduced the change even though a cereal-based menu constituted but a fraction of their habitual dietary choices.

The preference of starches as the dietary foundation is the same worldwide. Unsurprisingly, people seem to love their carbs. Americans, for example, dutifully follow the macronutrient consumption advice. The Standard American Diet, with its 50/15/35 carb/protein/fat ratio, fits into the recommended 45-65/10-35/20-35 ranges. In fact, the carbohydrate consumption is 15% lower than the maximum limit. It's encouraging to know that with the copious amounts of pizza, fries, bread, corn, fruit, soft drinks, sugar, doughnuts, ice cream, cakes, and other sweet and starchy foods, there is still room in our carbohydrate allowance. Of course, while conforming to the macronutrient advice, there are some recommendations still unfulfilled by the standard diet. In short, it looks like we are almost there with our dietary choices. So why are we doing so terribly health-wise?

Chapter Nine

Fallacies

From the modern perspective, it is easy to under-appreciate our hunter-gatherer forefathers. One particular aspect of their existence in the wild is typically glossed over—namely, their food preparation (culinary) skills. We mostly think of our pre-farming ancestors as accomplished hunters and pickers of edible plants. Those skills definitely deserve our appreciation; however, as humans, we can't survive for long on raw meat and wild plants. We need to have our meals nutritious, chewable and digestible. That requires the transformation of killed game and wild vegetation into nutritionally dense sustenance. Having at one's disposal only stone and wooden tools, meal preparation was by no means easy for our ancestors. It is not always a simple task to gather wood and start a fire, not to mention flay and cut game meat for the meal; then the meat has to be carefully baked or roasted to have its nutritional value enhanced and to render it easier to digest. A similar level of involvement is required when preparing plant-based dishes— it involves cutting and picking out seeds and any excessively fibrous or toxic parts. The idyllic view of the hunter-gatherers easily living off nutritious, easily accessible foods is a fantasy. Almost all the plant foods we eat raw today used to be scrawny, fibrous, and not very tasty. The precursors of our fruits and veggies were completely different than their modern equivalents. We have selectively cultivated our crops over millennia to suit our palates and digestive systems. That selective farming led to the transformation of wild plants into today's nourishing, easily digestible equivalents.

As the hunter-gatherers' digestive systems were virtually the same as ours are now, they had to significantly adapt their barely edible or inedible-in-raw-form plants before consumption. Therefore, they had a choice between either meat acquisition, which was risky and unpredictable but required less processing; or significantly labor-intensive plant food gathering and preparation. To increase their odds, they could have done both simultaneously. The men would hunt while the women and children would gather and prepare plant-based meals. Finding adequate vegetation and preparing it must have required specialized plant knowledge and cooking skills. In my view, the idealized image of our predecessors' easy living by picking plant foods, eating them immediately and spending most of the day relaxing is unrealistic. I've read many opinions about how the farming revolution ruined the happy-go-lucky lifestyle of the hunter-gatherers. I have a different take on the subject. Human existence has been always precarious and almost never effortless. The farmers were toiling on their land, unsure if their crops would fail due to the weather or pest invasion. The hunter-gatherers risked their lives hunting and worked hard preparing their meals, never knowing what to expect in the new hunting/foraging area. As the farmer's life was more structured and predictable, the nomadic life of their predecessors, while it followed some routine, relied more on daily improvisation. However, both required significant effort and specialized knowledge. Therefore, easy living off of the abundant hunting grounds and Garden-of-Eden-like foraging areas, while occasionally possible for hunter-gatherers, was most likely not the norm. Otherwise, why would they start farming?

Let's narrow our focus on the gatherer "easy living" fallacy. Disregarding today's farmed fruits and vegetables, only relatively few of them in their wild-grown forms qualify as directly consumable by humans. Some individuals even have problems digesting our cultivated veggies in their raw form; experiencing stomach cramps from consumption of raw cauliflower, broccoli, or even lettuce is not that uncommon. Now imagine how most of the wild-grown vegetation would affect our stomachs in its raw form. Herbivores can live on it because they have specialized, lengthy digestive systems perfectly suited to handle the highly-concentrated fiber contained in most plants. We don't. Our teeth and digestion call for more refined sustenance.

In fact, we are neither herbivores nor carnivores, nor even omnivores like the rest of the animals. Our ancestors used to pick the best parts of plants or game and then dice, mash, cook, ferment, dry, hydrate, or otherwise prepare them for eating. Our digestion is optimized for more nutritious and easier-to-digest sustenance than that directly available in nature. Our brains have evolved to require the consumption of meals which are nutritionally very dense. Thus, external food processing prior to digestion is built into our normal feeding routine. It might be argued that our food preparation skills have grown in proportion with our brains; the more we refined our sustenance, the more our brains developed, and vice versa. Therefore, the significant degree of food processing could be considered a major differentiating factor between us and the other animals, comparable to our advanced use of tools.

1.

Herbivore

Plants   Animals

2.

Carnivore

Plants   Animals

3.

Omnivore

Plants   Animals

Human

4.

Processing

Plants   Animals

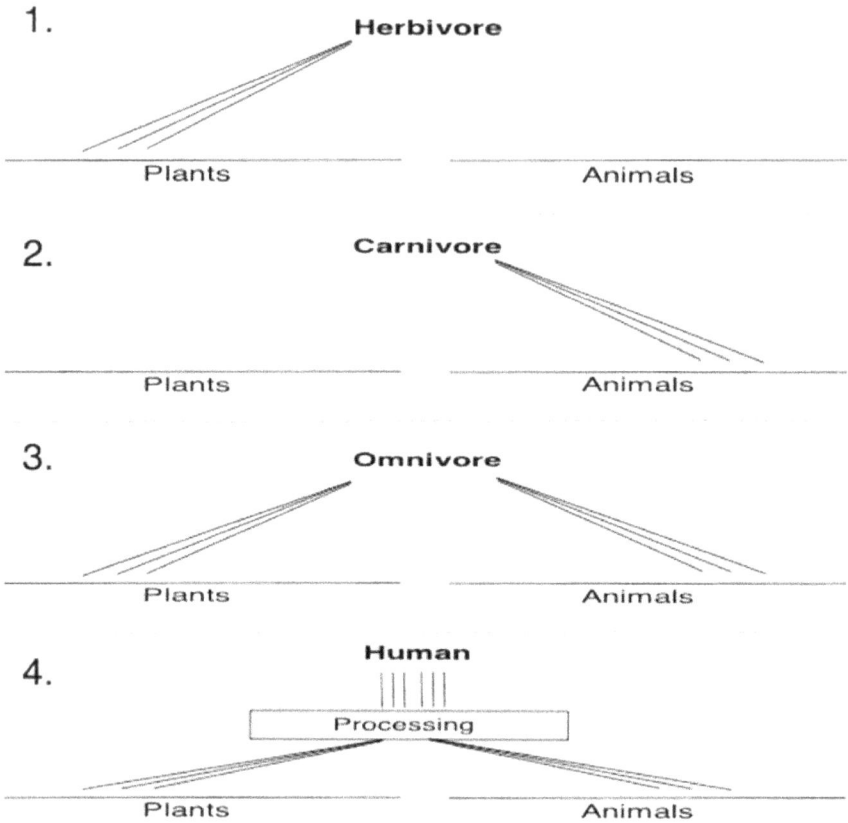

**Figure 5 - Human Eating Adaptation - compared
to other animals**

Adding to the difficulty of hunting and food preparation was our necessarily nomadic way of life. As foraging areas or hunting grounds became depleted, clans and tribes had to move to find new areas capable of supporting their living.

To sum it up, it's reasonable to assume that our ancestors seldom ate their foods unprepared; typically, they processed their plant and animal foods to increase chewability, digestibility, and nutrition. That thorough preparation resulted in more satisfying meals but required time and effort. From catching game animals or gathering plants, through the cleaning and separation of the most nutritious parts, and finally to cooking, our ancestors had to work hard for their meals. And having limited options for saving leftovers, they had to go almost daily through the extensive food procurement process. Thus, the assumption of the daily meal consolidation seems to make the most sense; which means that, after the meal was finally prepared, our forefathers probably partook in a sizeable feast later in the day. How late they dined depended on the time required to prepare the meal.

One notable fallacy is the belief in the extraordinary powers of frequent, high-dose vitamin supplementation. As previously mentioned, our bodies buffer vitamins and regulate their assimilation according to many factors. Think about how the Stone Age people were taking their vital nutrients—at random intervals, as contained in their meals. Today we assume that regular high-dose vitamin consumption is of great benefit. While it's probably not very harmful, neither is it optimal. When our pee turns fluorescent yellow after ingesting a mega-dose of vitamins, that's our body telling us where the extra vitamins should go. Our bodies expel additional vitamins like they do toxins.

Let's consider how vitamins naturally find their way to our bodies.

The most unusual of them is vitamin D. That essential substance is produced by our bodies as a response to sunshine hitting our skin. There is an optimal range of that vitamin, as it depends on the sun's exposure and the darkness of our skin. The darker the skin, the less vitamin D is produced. People living further from the equator developed lighter skin color to make up for the lesser sun exposure. However, to protect itself from overexposure to sunshine, our skin automatically darkens. Therefore, our level of vitamin D is limited by tanning and varies with our sun exposure, which in pre-civilizational reality would be proportional to our level of activity, as being busy indoors was not common for our ancestors. However, nowadays we work mostly inside or in the shade, so we should definitely boost our vitamin D level based on our activity level.

As is the case with vitamin D, our progenitors were supplied with other vitamins unevenly throughout the year. The frequency and dosage of those depended on the consumption of various foods during different seasons and from one foraging area to another. Thus, in the colder months, they ingested more meat-sourced vitamin combinations. In the warmer months, vegetation consumption would change the available vitamin assortment accordingly. Naturally, fasting periods would contribute to the irregularity of vitamin ingestion. It's important to note that intake doesn't equal internal availability; we stock the vitamins we need long-term together with the energy reserves in our body fat. These vitamins are fat-soluble. The other vitamins that stay in our body for a shorter time are water-soluble. It looks like we are "designed" to handle the fluctuation of water-soluble vitamin intake better than the fat-soluble vitamins that we have to carry on us all the time. Therefore, perhaps occasional scarcity of water-soluble vitamins is as optimal as it used to be unavoidable.

It's worth pointing out one big problem with modern dietary studies. They examine our nutrition using the eating pattern that doesn't fit our primal eating schedule. Notably, they are conducted with subjects eating three meals daily. That is an arbitrary consumption plan we have propagated since the advent of farming. As indicated earlier in this book, that schedule of eating is unsuitable for us. Compelling the participants to eat so frequently distorts the results of any given fixed-macronutrient diet studies. In other words, by eating constantly, we overload our digestive system—regardless of the specific foods we eat. Thus, performing studies with this factor as a common denominator is equivalent to comparing which anomaly is possibly less harmful.

A common misconception is that the human lifespan, which is much longer than our kin the apes', is purely accidental; that there is no survival benefit to our longevity. In other words, human life beyond the age of about forty is useless from the evolutionary perspective. On the face of it, when looking at us the same way as other animals, that statement makes sense. Once our children themselves reach the procreation age, we should be redundant, since they can now have their own children. However, consider our principal advantage over the rest of the animal kingdom—our intellect. To our ancestors, the elders were precious. They were like computers or encyclopedias. To a clan struggling for survival in the wild, the access to the knowledge and experience of seniors presented an enormous advantage. In addition to passing along practical survival knowledge and aiding in decision-making, the elders participated in raising and educating the children.

We don't spend much time considering this point, but the primitive (from our point of view) technology they used and the social structure of which they were members were quite intricate. As relatively crude as their know-how was, human societies have always been information-driven. Our advantage has been reliance on the mind much more than on the muscles and teeth. Think about the scope of the problems our nomadic ancestors had to cope with. They had to know everything concerning survival and social interactions: They were familiar with the terrain and knew how to heal wounds and make a fire, tools, weapons, and shelters; which foods were edible and how to prepare them; various hunting and fishing techniques; customs of behavior when encountering strangers; and the rules imposed on clan members and inter-clan exchanges. Our ancestors' very lives were dependent on their small daily decisions, more than ours are, and all the knowledge they possessed was contained in their heads. They had to think abstractly, remember facts, estimate, guess, plan, and so forth, with no aids other than each other. In that context, our ancestors' elders were indispensable. Therefore, the groups with the smarter, longer-living elders were in a much better position to survive.

Our longevity is no stroke of luck; we have evolved to age gracefully while exercising our mental and physical potential for the longest possible time. With the modern ways of passing knowledge in various forms and the narrow specializations individuals tend to develop, we don't rely on our elders the same way. It is mostly emotional bonds that connect us with our parents and grandparents. Therefore, their loss of mobility or intellectual capacity does not influence us in the same dramatic way as it would otherwise; it doesn't affect our survival. However, we should remember that it's not evolutionary programming that makes our elders into infirm, passive members of society. It's our suboptimal lifestyle that is at fault. And that includes its most significant contributor—nutrition.

According to the official nutritional guide we need fiber in our diet, as it's necessary to maintain the right balance of microorganisms in our gut. I have no doubt that is true. However, a question comes to mind: Where does the fiber come from when our menu switches to meat? The nutritional guide doesn't address that question, as it refers only to the high-carbohydrate diet. So maybe the statement should read: "To promote healthy gut flora, when eating carbohydrates we need to maintain a certain minimum amount of fiber in our diet." We don't need fiber to maintain our gut flora when eating like carnivores. That is interesting, considering that eating meat is a big part of our natural human diet.

We know that our pre-farming predecessors were consuming meat for most of the year. So maybe the main problem with our gut bacteria is the high concentration of carbohydrates when consumed in refined form. In that context, fiber's main role is to dilute the concentration of carbs in order to prevent starch-feeding bacteria from dominating our gut flora.

Salads typically supply a lot of fiber. We consider eating them a healthy junk food replacement. However, how much of the health benefit is related to the vitamins in the consumed greens and how much to the simple carbohydrate reduction? I'd say that beyond the necessary minuscule amounts, we simply don't need the extra vitamins and minerals. However, we unquestionably need the extra fiber to reduce the concentration of starches in the gut.

Our body chemistry and microbiota surrounding us are heavily dependent on our long-term diet. As we age, the body can't handle the constant flow of starches. Picture a pasta pot boiling over with bubbling goo spilling down the sides. That is how our body reacts to the relentless flow of carb-y sustenance. With the steady influx of refined carbs, our skin microbe mix changes similarly to how our gut flora does. While the body tries to keep up with the incoming starches, its auto-regulating functions lose their effectiveness. Our sweat and sebaceous glands secrete too much or too little of the chemically altered excretions. That allows hostile microorganisms to take hold of our skin.

The smell of our bodies, or the absence of smell, depends on the composition of our sweat and sebum and the type of microbes prevailing on our skin. Those microbes break down our shedding skin and its shielding secretions, releasing different odors in the process. The right chemical composition of our bodily excretions, along with the proper functioning of our defense mechanisms, should keep the skin surface chemistry and microorganisms within a proper neutral range. Thus, with the appropriate diet, our skin should not smell offensively, nor should it require frequent washing and application of odor-masking or hydrating or dehydrating lotions. Think about it. The body auto-regulates itself to a tremendous degree, including lubricating the skin and balancing its microbial colonies. And yet we have to help it by getting rid of the natural protection and replacing it with the "improved" versions of our own invention?

The arbitrary ways in which we nourish ourselves and then deal with the outcomes are a part of a larger illogical pattern. In many cases, we ignore our adaptation to nature. We go against it and are surprised by the consequences. Consider our approach to vitamins. It's true that before enriching white flour, there were many cases of vitamin deficiency; however, after partially fixing that problem by adding the vitamins back into the flour and fortifying milk with vitamin D, most adults started getting enough vitamins from their diet. Except for one—vitamin D. We became aware of that deficiency upon seeing children develop rickets. Therefore, we started giving young children vitamin D supplements. That decision again presumably solved the vitamin deficiency problem.

However, we are aware that most of us still lack vitamin D. To come to that conclusion required extensive scientific studies. Researchers established that there are many risk factors for having the deficiency. Here are some of them:

- Poverty
- Obesity
- Gender (girls are more likely to be deficient)
- Television, video game, and/or computer use of more than four hours per day
- Milk consumption less than once a day
- Age (older children/adolescents are more often deficient)
- Darker skin

Also, a lack of vitamin D is associated with a wide range of afflictions, from certain cancers to common back pain.

Let's consider that for a moment. We know that our ancestors were getting loads of vitamin D independently of what they ate, by mere sun exposure. Since we stay inside most of the time and put sunscreen on when we do go outside, how can we get enough of that vital substance? We would have to consume foods like fish or specific processed, enriched foods in large quantities to get us to a satisfactory vitamin D level. We can ask ourselves this question: If we can get that vitamin from food, why don't our bodies rely on that method exclusively? Why the reliance on sun exposure? That method of vitamin D dosage makes its delivery activity-dependent instead of relying exclusively on nutrition. That method of "supply" works the same way for all of us, yet we recommend supplementation to only specific groups of people at specific stages of life. Why? The logical thing would be to assume that all of us need as much of that vitamin as our nomadic predecessors. As with the proper diet, adequate levels of vitamin D should be a starting point of healthy living.

Let's look at another example of focusing on treatments while neglecting prevention.

We know that our jaws are underdeveloped. They can't accommodate all our teeth. Look at the lower jaws of the people around you. Many of them have an overbite and crooked teeth. That is the typical look of modern people in the industrialized world. To remedy that, as adults, we need to have our wisdom teeth removed. Also, a great number of us straighten out the crooked teeth in childhood or later in life. Everybody knows about this problem. And we know that it's not an evolutionary accident. Aboriginal people's teeth are straight and evenly spaced. We should also have developed that way. Our lower jaw should be more prominent and our bite even. The American Association of Orthodontists (AAO) estimates that 75%

of Americans suffer from an improper bite and could benefit from orthodontic treatment.

It's our diet that causes the abnormality. Most likely it is vitamin deficiency which doesn't manifest otherwise, combined with the soft foods that we eat as children, that causes this deformation. The best way to fix it would be to find out exactly what's wrong and recommend the proper preventive measures. Those could be more vitamins plus firmer foods for children. Instead, as with other aspects of our nutrition, rather than fix the diet, we rely on remedies. The attitude boils down to this: Let children have small jaws and crooked teeth; we can fix some of it later with oral surgery and orthodontia. In fact, we put lots of effort and money into developing state-of-the-art orthodontics and oral surgery options. The two would be very obscure disciplines if we were to place the emphasis instead on prevention.

In general, our approach is to use preventive measures only to stop extreme cases like rickets or other severe consequences of our unnatural lifestyle. We go the prevention route when we can establish a clear link between a deficiency and its effects to a very high degree of certainty. The following question comes to mind: What if many of the anomalies happening in our body due to a deficit are too complex or take too long to manifest for us to determine causality? Should we wait until we conduct enough research to widen our recommendations as we discover more risk factors? Or, perhaps, we should consider humans' natural environment as the necessary precondition to healthy living and use that as the baseline of our health assessment.

Chapter Ten

How Our Diet Fails

Many pundits insist that our calorie intake should closely match our energy expenditure. It's a reasonable-sounding proposition, but how feasible is it for us in our current circumstances? As indicated in previous chapters, the balancing of our calories is very difficult in our current nutritional environment. If we had evolved in the conditions of a steady food supply, that balance shouldn't be a problem. We should be able to overeat and discard the extra ingested calories instead of storing it as fat. Returning to reality, however, we have to recognize that, like every other animal on the planet, we evolved to survive with an irregular food supply. And, like other mammals, we have an energy-buffering scheme to store and retrieve it according to nourishment availability and our activity level.

Let's compare the energy balancing of the human body to the buffering function of a rechargeable battery. For starters, let's define some terms. Regarding the battery's operation, the word "cycle" denotes the period needed to charge a unit to 100% and drain it back to zero. In reality, the battery is rarely fully discharged. However, the total operational time of charging and discharging can be divided by the duration of one full charge-and-discharge cycle. That figure is the number of cycles the battery went through, and is a good predictor of the battery's lifespan. In fact, it is better than just the age of the unit. Let's say that a battery is designed to handle two thousand cycles. It doesn't matter if the battery goes through those cycles in one year or five; after those two thousand cycles, the battery wears out and is no longer functional.

What if we, as biological machines, have an equivalent wear component? That means that our digestive systems and metabolism carry a limit of useful cycles.

Taking the battery analogy even further, we can look at another significant form of premature wear-down: *how* we cycle the battery. Batteries are designed for so-called shallow and deep cycles. Depending on the amount of the drainage, the battery may be depleted only minimally (shallow cycle) or to a significant degree (deep cycle) before recharging. For example, the car battery is designed to shallow-cycle. This means that its operation is optimal when the battery is only slightly discharged and almost constantly charged. In contrast to that, emergency power backup batteries fare much better with nearly complete depletions. If one were to use the car battery for backup, its useful number of cycles would be reduced. The same significant shortening of useful cycles occurs when using a deep-cycle battery for shallow-cycle application. In other words, nothing is stopping us from using those batteries interchangeably, but if we decide to do it, we must be aware that their lifespan will be severely compromised.

Having that deep- and shallow-cycling idea in mind, let's return to the human metabolic battery. Our eating of three meals a day plus snacks is equivalent to the shallow-battery cycles. In that scenario, we use our energy (discharge) while eating throughout the day (charge). That concurrency and the fact of the shallow energy expenditure before recharging presents a radically different pattern than that we've evolved to follow. Our predecessors did not have foods within their reach. Before eating, they had to obtain and prepare their food. Thus, they significantly discharged their metabolic battery by hunting and cooking before being able to recharge it by participating in the afternoon or evening feast.

Our bodies are more sophisticated than a simple battery, however; they have a few different metabolic buffers.

The most accessible energy reserve is glycogen. This is conveniently packaged glucose that can be released into the bloodstream depending on our energy expenditure. That reserve is sufficient for many hours of activity.

The slightly less accessible but much more abundant energy reserves we carry are fats. Those fat-derived energy transports are called fatty acids and triglycerides. Like glucose, we have a supply of these in our bloodstream and liver, as well as abundant stocks in our fat cells. Using those different reserves allowed our ancestors to function independently of the irregular food supply. It was the way their bodies operated for hundreds of thousands of years.

Let's compare the two eating patterns. The graphs below compare the energy supply and expenditure of our modern and original consumption models.

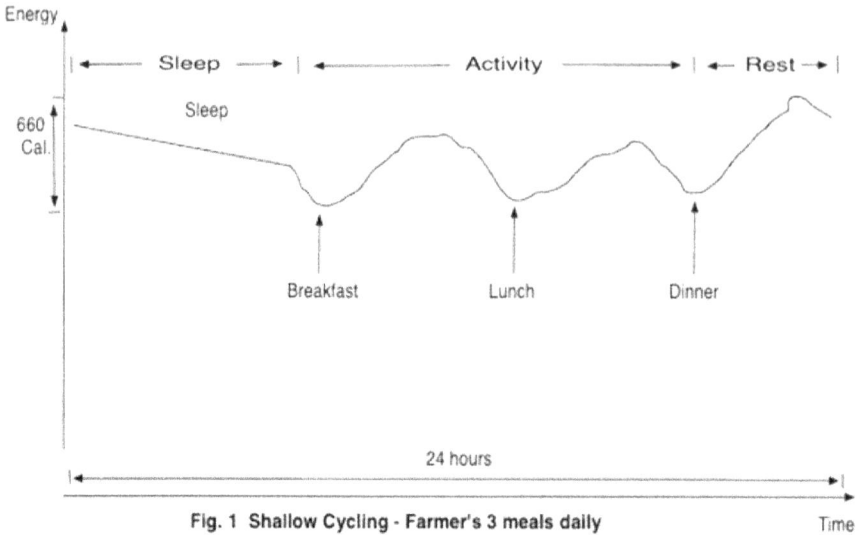

Fig. 1 Shallow Cycling - Farmer's 3 meals daily

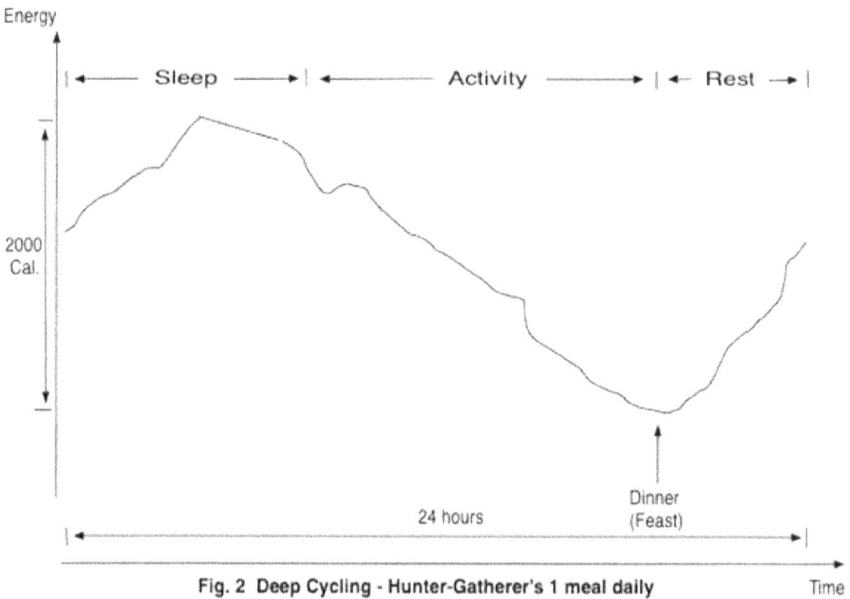

Fig. 2 Deep Cycling - Hunter-Gatherer's 1 meal daily

Figure 1 illustrates our current plan for three meals daily. Note that we re-supply ourselves with energy throughout the day. Other than while we are sleeping, the entirety of our digestive system operates constantly.

Figure 2 shows an example of the optimal plan of one meal daily. In it, our energy is depleted significantly before the meal. Of course, the timing of the meal may vary; however, the long fasting time indicated by the downward slope brings about the steady energy supply state which is natural to our species.

Our three carb-filled meals daily plus snacking bypasses that buffering mechanism, delivering glucose from quickly assimilating starchy foods directly to the bloodstream. Due to the quite rapid absorption, this type of delivery causes the glucose supply to be uneven.

Over the last few thousand years, we started disregarding that sophisticated buffering adaptation. Instead, we fill our stomachs frequently and make our digestion work continually throughout the day.

Another problem with the current dietary practice is the insistence on the fixed macronutrient ratio. What makes matters worse is that the ratio of the nutrients recommended is one that would be rare for our nomadic ancestors, as high-carbohydrate foods were quite a rarity before the farming revolution.

Supplying our body with nutrients is a very involved operation. Let's imagine our gastrointestinal tract and metabolic system to be a complex food-processing factory. Designed to be efficient and auto-regulating within a wide margin, its task is to take in a wide range of foods and convert them into specific body fuels. Depending on the macronutrient profile of the incoming food, different fuels are produced. When carbohydrate-rich food is being supplied, the factory breaks it easily into glucose—fuel number one. On the receiving end, when the blood glucose is low, more of it is added directly from the factory. Any remaining glucose is used to replenish the immediate reserves (glycogen stores in the liver and muscles). After the reserves are full, the surplus is converted to fat and put away in cells for long-term storage.

If starch intake in the incoming food drops, the body starts utilizing different fuels. And thus, more fats (fuel number two) are being used by the muscles and the precious glucose from the carbohydrates is designated for the brain. When the starch content drops lower still, glucose for the brain is supplemented by the glucose newly generated by the liver. When there are practically no carbohydrates coming in, the body switches to an alternative fuel: the ketones, fuel number three. Ketones are the chemicals synthesized in the liver from the available fat. Whereas all three fuels may be used by most of the body, the brain can only utilize glucose and ketones. The conversion from glucose to ketones is a hard one for us because it affects our brain. However, fueling with ketones may have its benefits, and that switch was natural to our ancestors. We are unsure whether not going into ketosis for at least part of the year doesn't compromise our long-term health, especially our mental health.

The preceding image of body fueling is obviously simplified. The point here is that the flexibility of our digestive and metabolic system working in conjunction with the rest of the body is astonishing. We can ingest foods in different combinations and the body adjusts its operation accordingly, in that it uses short- and long-term reserves and switches between different fuels. In its fueling flexibility, different parts of the digestive tract and metabolic paths are used. What that means is that some organs or parts of the organs rest or regenerate while the others take over the heavy lifting. With a steady high-carbohydrate diet, we wear out our carbohydrate path by using it all the time. We know hunter-gatherers consumed starchy foods much less often than we do. They were relying mostly on meat for their survival. Even if we assume that they moved between the fats, proteins, and carbs with equal frequency (each a third of the time), we can see the tremendous difference between our ancestors' and our utilization of the digestive/metabolic system.

Like our ancestors, we may need to periodically switch our foods to exercise all digestive/metabolic paths for our general health. The intention here is not only to ensure that we do not overtax various organs. The significant variations in nutritional content, including periodic eating abstention and the associated hormonal shifts, may be of tremendous significance for overall, long-term well-being. If you're not convinced about our diet-switching adaptation, try imagining yourself living in the wild. Look around a forest or meadow and try to assess the nutritional qualities of whatever vegetation is growing around you. Ask yourself how much effort it would require to gather those tiny wild seeds and scrawny wild fruits. Even if you located a place with densely growing edible plants, how long would they last if they had to feed a whole group of people? What guarantee do you have that you would find another bountiful source of food nearby to replace this one immediately after you've exhausted it? How long would you have to walk to find another one? Remember that our energy requirements are significant, and the hunter-gatherers tended to roam in groups. The groups included children, pregnant women, and the elderly, who were unable to contribute much to the food-acquiring efforts.

What solution was there to these problems in that era of human history? In general, you ate what you were able to get and as much as you could. You had to switch your foods based on what was available. Since most of the available plants were not very nutritious, as well as difficult to chew and digest, you adapted them by appropriate processing. Once you learned how to prepare your meals, there was a wide array of food sources at your disposal. However, they may have varied significantly depending on the weather, the season, and the hunting/foraging region. Therefore, if you didn't catch that animal and a fruit was available, you went for the latter. If a starchy root vegetable or a mushroom was growing, you cooked and ate it. If there was a river nearby, you tried to catch fish. If you found edible insects, you also appreciated them as a good nutrition source. That way, you easily went from one day to another between starchy roots, meats, leafy greens, fruits, and nuts. Yes, most of them required some work to catch or gather and make edible, but that was no big problem. You were a human and that's what you did. You improved your foods; you were not completely at the mercy of nature, like other animals. You switched up your nourishment because you didn't have a choice. However, you figured out how to make it suitable for you. Sometimes, when you had abundant caloric food sources, you instinctively overate. Other times, when you couldn't catch or find anything, you just didn't eat. For a long time, our nomadic predecessors were in the position of being half in control of their sustenance and half at the mercy of nature. Admittedly, this had to have been much better than the situation of other animals that could not adapt as quickly to various nutritional environments.

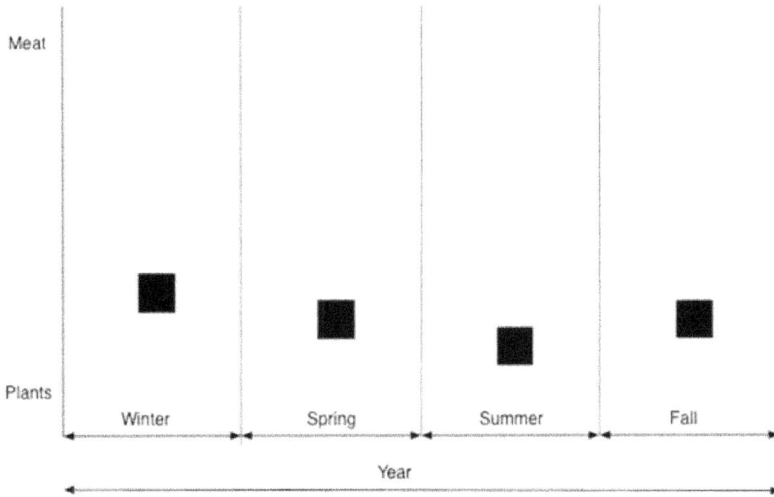

Fig. 3 . Meat vs. Plants - Modern Diet

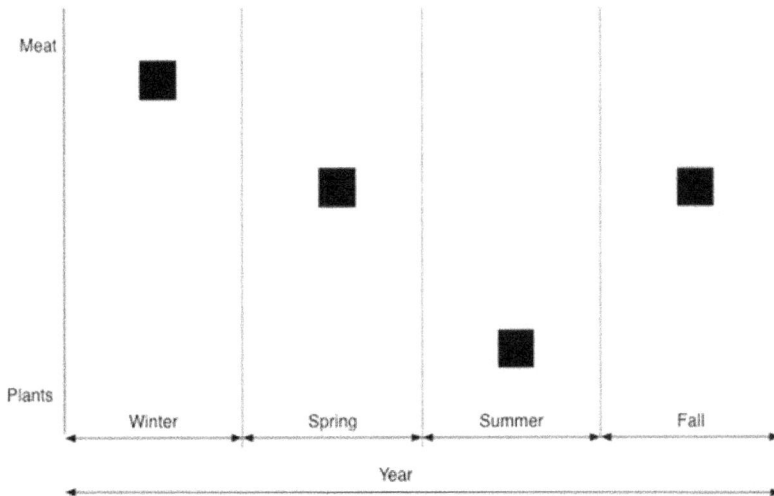

Fig. 4 Meat vs. Plants - Early Human Diet

Figures 3 and 4 illustrate the difference in diversity between us and the early humans. Obviously, they don't represent a comparison of any specific diets. They indicate that hunter-gatherers were able and most of the time compelled to radically switch up their menu. Please note that nowadays, plant-sourced proteins might be a good substitute for meat; however, for our predecessors, meat was a very practical and universally available sustenance.

Let's go back to the food-processing factory analogy. From our mouth to the large intestine, incoming food is processed mechanically and chemically to break it down and extract the maximum number of nutrients while moving toxins and unnecessary material along to be eventually expelled. The timing of every stage of the processing is dependent on many factors. One of them is how quickly nutrients can be absorbed and possibly further processed. Thus, depending on the content of the incoming food, nutrients are absorbed in different places at different rates. Therefore, the flow of the sustenance slows down and speeds up based on many factors. The system is designed to have one portion of food loaded and devote the remainder of the day to performing its full digestive cycle. Therefore, a steady food supply may have some negative consequences. In general, it rushes the processing, thereby potentially compromising the thoroughness of preprocessing and the efficiency of the assimilation. Another issue is that since the upper gastrointestinal tract works quite fast, it should stay idle for many hours. The mouth, esophagus, and stomach should be resting almost all the time. Eating over the twelve-hour period shortens that recuperation period significantly.

Now, if we consume refined carbohydrates, the back end of the glucose assimilation system can be severely overloaded. Sometimes, it just can't keep up with the incoming starches. Therefore, the line slows down. As the concentrated carbohydrates stay longer in our intestines, they create a perfect opportunity for microorganisms to feast. The carb-overloaded moist and warm intestine is the ideal petri dish for all kinds of not-so-friendly microbes. Keeping in mind the vast surface area of our guts, we can imagine the stress to our body when combatting that microbial army on such a long frontline. The intestine also needs a periodic rest—not as frequently as the upper gastrointestinal tract, but once in a while it needs a complete shutdown. That is one reason we require occasional fasting.

Let's take another look at our eating frequency.

There are cues our body sends to our brain which hint at what it expects from us. For example, we receive a not-so-subtle clue as to what should happen after a sufficiently sumptuous meal—we get sluggish and drowsy. That seems to suggest that the digestion should ideally be undisturbed and occur when we are inactive, like when we sleep. On the flip side, alertness coincides with an empty stomach. Thus, when we fast during the day, our brain is not affected by the hormonal processes related to digestion but fully concentrated on supporting our daily ventures. The same applies to physical activity. We know that we shouldn't swim, run, or engage in other strenuous activities immediately after a meal. It just makes sense. So why do we eat throughout the day?

At this point, let's return to the issue of hunger. As many proudly proclaim, we have mostly eliminated it in industrialized societies. I am aware that the slogan "to eliminate hunger" is in fact meant to imply "to eradicate malnutrition." However, in reality, through our farm-era eating pattern, we have mostly suppressed hunger related to the replenishing of our energy reserves. That brought to the forefront a similar feeling—hunger related to stockpiling extra energy. That is because we experience that same powerful eating compulsion, but for different reasons. Since the perception is the same, however, it's difficult for us to distinguish between different cravings. And because they are so closely related to our survival, we respond to them the way we are supposed to: We obey them.

The brain urges us to eat for two reasons. The first craving is triggered when we run out of stored calories. Let's call that one "survival hunger." The second one manifests when the brain senses the opportunity of acquiring extra calories from an especially nutritious meal. Let's call that one "binge hunger." The first one hardly requires a comment since that is our primary motivator to eat. The second, the binge signal, can also be quite strong. It only occurs when consuming suitably compelling meals, and it readily overrides our feeling of fullness.

Contributors to the obesity epidemic are the eradication of survival hunger and the cultivation of binge hunger. The recommended eating-throughout-the-day routine takes care of the first kind. We don't even have a chance to experience it, as we start munching early in the morning and continue until late in the evening. The second kind of hunger, however, flourishes due to the primal lure and frequent consumption of highly-caloric meals. Who doesn't experience that craving for an additional slice of pizza, a slice of cake, or an extra portion of fries? That hunger mix-up is the curse of modern society. As per our "design," we should regularly experience survival hunger and rarely feel binge hunger. The feeling of hunger after a fasting period is natural, and its higher intensity should be our signal to start eating. The key here is the level of craving. If we were accustomed to that sensation, as our forefathers were, we would completely disregard it when experiencing it in its gentle form. We would go about our lives distracted easily by the tasks at hand. The proper interpretation of the mild post-fast craving is: "I am ready to eat." One might be surprised to find out how long it takes even for that subtle feeling to manifest.

The term "breakfast" refers literally to the breaking of the nightly fast. When we sleep, we are abstaining from food, but that is hardly an intentional state. And, for most of us, that is the only period in which we don't eat. However, in the morning we start eating automatically. That is a big mistake. We should start eating differently. That is, only if we are hungry—not when prompted by a clock. Clearly, when we get hungry depends on the size and the caloric value of the prior meal, as well as on our energy expenditure. However, when the last meal was sufficiently caloric and our activity level is moderate, the food craving appears only after quite a long time. In our deep-charging battery analogy, that is the period needed for the metabolic system to complete discharging and become ready for recharging. It also gives our digestive system the opportunity to complete its full digestion cycle undisturbed. The farming-era-invented breakfast, as unnatural as it is, could have been introduced for practical reasons. In anticipation of an exhausting work day, it was thought prudent to overload our digestive system to prepare our energy store for the time that we would "run out of fuel." In that way, in theory, we could lessen, or even avoid, hunger and related distractions. However, there are two issues with that approach. The first is that we already have the reserve of energy at our disposal that should be used before refueling. The second is that refueling during the day has even more of an impact on productivity. Although we are not fully aware of it, our body after breakfast is working hard at processing the meal. Thus we experience physical manifestations of digestion plus a series of attention fluctuations induced by changes in blood sugar levels. Those waves of drowsiness and buzz make us uncomfortable. To steady things out, we reach for snacks and caffeine.

Preventive ingestion is a misguided "improvement" introduced by farmers. We should be relying on the body's eating-encouragement prompts and its capacity to supply glucose, triglycerides, or ketones steadily to our organs. High-carbohydrate snacks are the unquestionable favorite. Consuming them will energize us but will also result in craving when the stimulus ceases. Where do we see that pattern of periodically reaching for stimulants and experiencing the highs followed by the inevitable lows? In other types of addictions.

Of course, these foods exert a powerful influence on our mind. Sugars and other carbohydrates, due to their quick metabolizing, increase the amplitude of the mood fluctuations. That is another reason we should avoid eating them on a whim—they are as bad for our body as they are dangerous to our mind. The mechanism and individual susceptibility to the mood-altering powers of nutrition are quite apparent. Our varying sensitivity to it, however, is often responsible for our not fully realizing the gravity of the problem. Some individuals don't have significantly strong food cravings. Their brain-metabolic system connection is not as powerful. But for others, I would argue most of us, it's quite the opposite. And yet we promote and advertise food as if it were furniture. I take that back—food sales are much more aggressive. Add to that the cultural and social pressures plus the neutral government policy, and the recipe for the nutritional pathology is complete.

Let's make this point clear: Eating ahead of time to avoid the feeling of hunger is another one of those occasions when our conscious mind overrides our instincts. Which one should we follow, the hunger directive from our metabolic system or our conscious decision based on the simplistic comprehension of our body "fueling"?

When it has sufficient energy reserves, the body functions optimally in a fasted state—a condition in which, absent the considerable exertion required by digestion, it can focus on regulating its functions and fighting infections. In extreme cases, the body sends a powerful signal to our mind, telling us to abstain from eating.

We all experience the body's attempt at shutting down the digestive system. For example, have you noticed the first thing that happens when we get sick? With incoming fever we often immediately lose our appetite. And it's not a mild disinterest in food; in that state of illness, it becomes difficult to force ourselves to eat even small amounts.

That's our body clearly signaling our mind to avoid eating so that it can focus entirely on fighting the illness. Unfortunately, many of our caretakers try to second-guess that reaction; they try to make us eat, reasoning that with our belly full of food, we will have more strength to fight the illness. That otherwise common-sense thinking is wrong because it contradicts our body's explicit request.

Why is it so difficult to understand that we should obey our body's hunger and thirst signals? After all, we follow the body's signaling on when to use the restroom. In fact, we are strongly discouraged by health professionals to force or delay our restroom visits. So why should we eat and drink according to a schedule? Our digestion and metabolism are not that transparent. The time necessary to process and assimilate foods varies. The processing may slow down or speed up depending on the fiber content and macronutrient ratios of our meals.

Additionally, it can be affected by other processes occurring within the body. The metabolism undergoes similar rules; it's flexible. It varies from individual to individual and, among other factors, it depends on the proportions of muscle, fat, and age. In short, it is a complicated process.

We have the feeling of hunger for a purpose. It's a signal that our readily available energy reserve is low. Note that we are talking about *readily available* energy; our total reserve lasts typically about a month. Let's compare that to the status of a car's fuel gauge. In that scenario, the equivalent of the hunger signal would appear as the needle moving about one-thirtieth of the full range. The change would be hardly noticeable. But that slightly paranoid urge to replenish our energy reserve has its justification: Our body doesn't want to dip into its long-term reserves. Therefore, it sends us the quite strong eating-encouragement signal. Our ancestors would get this signal normally once a day and it would coincide with the readiness of their meal. It's important to react to that prototypical call-to-meal rather than preempt it! Unfortunately, the three-daily-meals routine is doing exactly that. It's forcing the extra work on our unprepared digestive and metabolic systems.

All other animals listen to their hunger signal—and so should we. We haven't evolved enough in the last few thousand years to be able to bypass it without compromising our health. And yet we do it because we have food within our reach. It's a perfect example of our precocious brain sabotaging our well-being.

Here is the crux of the matter: The pleasure/satisfaction signals are sent to the brain while we eat, even though we are not hungry. So it's enough for us to start eating—our natural feeding compulsion takes care of the rest.

It can't be stressed enough that eating triggers a significant food processing operation. When we ingest we don't magically inject glycogen into our muscles and liver. We engage our digestive system, and that has its consequences.

Digestion is a very involved process requiring the commitment of many bodily systems. There are hormones, enzymes, muscles, and multiple organs at work to process incoming food. It's demanding, and it shouldn't be undertaken casually.

Since hormones are heavily involved in the process of digestion, there are two distinctive hormonal states of our body. The first is the fasted state, optimized for activity, and the second is digestive, optimized for digestion. As we know, our whole body, including the brain and muscles, are influenced heavily by hormones. Therefore, by eating throughout the day in addition to overworking the digestion, we are making ourselves function in a suboptimal hormonal state. The fasted state should be our active state. That's the optimal setting to be in when exercising and engaging in intellectual activities. The digestive state is when we should rest and relax. That division is very natural, straightforward, and intuitive. So why do we hear the mantra about the health benefits of regular meal times?

Also, why do we have to make ourselves drink a certain number of glasses of water? Is that because of the meals that we have forced ourselves to eat? We should drink the same way we should eat—when prompted. Sipping steadily from a water bottle is not the way our ancestors satisfied their thirst. Water used to be a precious commodity; it wasn't always at hand. Most likely our ancestors settled down near water sources. However, when they were on the go, water was not readily available. It's not hard to imagine that they would occasionally spend a day or two without it. Our bodies are accustomed to automatically balancing their water stocks. After drinking, the body keeps enough of the precious fluid for quite some time. Notice that when we drink frequently, we are forcing our body to expel the extra water to maintain the fluid balance. Even when we sweat profusely, we do not always feel thirst immediately. Somehow, we have persuaded ourselves that this delayed reaction is a malfunction that needs to be rectified. Again, we second-guess our physiology.

Why do we do that? Mostly marketing. We associate healthy images with frequent hydration. Why exactly is sipping water during exercise healthy? Why do we have the urgency to replace the sweated-out water? Dehydration, like fasting, may be dangerous. However, the reason for it may be that our bodies are not accustomed to that natural state, more than anything else. Can you imagine our ancestors chasing animals while carrying a water container and stopping occasionally to take a sip? Again, with our simplistic understanding that more is somehow better, we are trying to "improve" our body's functioning but hindering its operation in the process. Maybe our gastrointestinal tract and kidneys should rest more and not be bothered by the constant flow of water?

Not listening to the physiological signaling of our body usually means making it work harder. Ordinarily, we should be thirsty when our body needs water. It's as simple as that. How unlikely is it that our body's hunger and thirst won't work for us? Very. Those signals are critical to our survival, and our body is optimized for using them on its own terms.

We must be aware of the degree of sophistication of our biological machine that we call the body. It auto-regulates itself without our awareness. And there is a purpose to that separation of concerns— it simplifies the operation by dividing the responsibilities. While our body and the inner parts of our brain work on maintaining our life functions, the conscious part of the brain is free to focus on solving the big-picture problems. That separation also builds an element of safety. Our conscious part of the brain is entirely free to think any kinds of thoughts and yet is incapable of accidentally stopping our breathing or our heartbeat.

We took advantage of that method of engineering a long time ago in building our computers. Most computing devices have at least those two levels of operation. There is the automatic, self-contained software directly controlling the hardware. We call that direct hardware link firmware, also known as BIOS in the personal computer world. Firmware is an equivalent of the innermost part of the brain which independently controls our vital life functions.

Then we have the operating system—Windows or macOS, to name the most common—which could be the equivalent of our conscious mind. The operating system runs different programs, just as our minds engage in various thought processes.

We can, of course, run different applications on our computers. However, they can't directly interfere with the firmware. That way we don't have to worry that a rogue program will crash the computer.

Similarly, our random thoughts operate independently from our breathing, digestion, and other essential life functions. That separation of responsibilities is super-important. The semi-independent operation of both subsystems, where they prompt each other for responses, is optimal. As our conscious mind is not interrupted by the minutiae of our heart, lung, liver, and kidney functions, we shouldn't barge in with our mind's decisions on the elaborate operation of our biological firmware. There is a proper communication channel between the two. It has been created and perfected by millions of years of evolution, and we should trust it. Through that channel, we get specific signals like pain, drowsiness, alertness, hunger, thirst, and satiety. Just listen to your body. It's a routinely ignored cliché, but it's the best summary of the way we ought to interact with it.

We know we can survive without food for multiple weeks. So why are we so paranoid about the slightest feeling of hunger? We should wait for it, as it is a reminder that our body is ready to take in more nutrition. Remember that we are talking here about survival-driven hunger. As discussed before, binge hunger will appear if we place ourselves in a situation in which the gorging stimuli fire up. Preparing that steaming pan of bacon and eggs with fresh bread and a glass of orange juice in the morning will certainly do the trick. It will make us binge-hungry instantaneously. We may expect a similar reaction when we visit a bakery, fast food place, doughnut shop, or ice cream parlor.

Now, let's look at some eating patterns that are gaining popularity recently among the brave dieting experimenters. They represent an alternative to the traditional three-meals-daily recommendation. Here they are:

Fasting: abstaining from food.

Dry Fasting: abstaining from food and drink.

One Meal A Day (OMAD): as the name suggests, eating one meal daily.

Intermittent fasting: restriction of the feeding window to a few hours.

Most dietitians and health professionals would discourage us from trying any of those ways of restricting our food intake. They would say that it's unhealthy. They have their reasons. Conditioned by decades of eating steadily through the day, we may react badly for a while to the sudden break of routine. That reaction should make us realize the extent of how different the two eating patterns are.

Here is the rub: All those supposedly harmful ways of eating are natural to our species and pretty much all animals on the planet.

Surviving in an environment where the food supply is unpredictable, one must undergo periods when sustenance is unavailable. Thus, fasting periods of varying duration, despite being an occasional nuisance, used to be a fact of life. What if, contrary to what health professionals think, the prolonged fasted state is beneficial? And, since it used to be unavoidable, it is vital for our periodic regeneration. All-day or multi-day food abstention is just an extension of our natural multi-hour fasting between meals.

Like the rest of the animal kingdom, our adaptation to periods of food scarcity may be a feature, not a bug, in our "design."

Here is the definition of fasting from Wikipedia[9]:

---

[9] **"Fasting."** *Wikipedia.* Accessed October 6, 2018. **https://en.wikipedia.org/wiki/Fasting**.

Fasting is the willing abstinence or reduction from some or all food, drink, or both, for a period of time. An absolute fast or dry fasting is normally defined as abstinence from all food and liquid for a defined period, usually 24 hours, or a number of days. Water fasting refers to abstinence from all food and drinks except water, but black coffee and tea may be consumed. Other fasts may be partially restrictive, limiting only particular foods or substances, or be intermittent. In a physiological context, fasting may refer to the metabolic status of a person who has not eaten overnight, or to the metabolic state achieved after complete digestion and absorption of a meal. Several metabolic adjustments occur during fasting.

Those metabolic adjustments affect, among other things, our hormonal system, and the promotion of autophagy,[10] both of which may be of crucial importance to our long-term health. Here is Wikipedia's definition of autophagy:

Autophagy [...] is the natural, regulated mechanism of the cell that disassembles unnecessary or dysfunctional components. Autophagy allows the orderly degradation and recycling of cellular components.

Below is an excerpt from Wikipedia concerning autophagy and caloric restriction [11].

---

[10] "**Autophagy.**" *Wikipedia.* Accessed October 7, 2018. **https://en.wikipedia.org/wiki/Autophagy.**
[11] "**Autophagy.**" *Wikipedia.* Accessed October 3, 2018. **https://en.wikipedia.org/wiki/Autophagy#Caloric_restriction.**

Research suggests that autophagy is required for the lifespan-prolonging effects of caloric restriction. A 2010 French study of nematodes, mice, and flies showed that inhibition of autophagy exposed cells to metabolic stress. Resveratrol and dietary restriction prolonged the lifespan of normal, autophagy-proficient nematodes, but not of nematodes in which autophagy had been inhibited by knocking out Beclin 1 (a known autophagic modulator).

So there we have it: a link between fasting (caloric restriction) and life extension. Of course, we should be careful about applying studies of simple organisms to the functioning of human bodies. However, if that link applies to us, which is very likely, we are losing a tremendous opportunity to naturally increase our lifespan.

Arguably, our bodies are better aligned with variability than steadiness of diet. It's hard to imagine Stone Age nomadic people having food supplies always at hand. Wasn't the lure of the idea of food stocks the reason they settled down and started farming in the first place?

Since we are still biologically those nomads, we are optimized for food intermittence and diversity, but not necessarily the variety promoted by today's nutrition guidelines, which is swapping one similar food for another, like different kinds of peppers, nuts, or fruits. The proper diet variation should be much more radical. Our original diet changed in its macronutrient ratio, fiber content, and quantity of sustenance. That is why all modern diets are suboptimal. They promote different but fixed macronutrient ratios. They can suit us in the short term; from the long-term perspective, however, consuming the same fat/protein/carbohydrate proportions over long periods of time is not optimal.

Let's return to the complex system analogy to show how nutrition influences our bodies.

It's important that the system operates within its optimal external parameter range. Can a system work in a suboptimal environment? Yes—if it's sophisticated enough, it can adjust itself to its external conditions. It can even cope with adverse circumstances. However, there are limits to that autoregulation. If the suboptimal conditions are too extreme or they exist for too long, the system will start failing prematurely.

Let's consider this. Our bodies can cope with toxic assaults of various kinds. For example, we may smoke or drink for many years until our lungs and liver get overwhelmed by the incoming toxins and lung cancer or liver cirrhosis develop. Also, we can function while consuming too little fiber in our carb-y diet for many years with compromised nutrient absorption and immune system. Medicines help with many conditions caused by improper eating. However, that "healing" which medication brings about is in fact just masking the underlying problem. It gives a false sense of security, as even with pharmacological crutches, there are limits to the continual suboptimal operation of our organs. And, obviously, they vary between individuals depending on many circumstances. However, improper nourishment catches up with us eventually. Diabetes type two is the name we assigned to the wearing down of the pancreas by carbohydrates. Also, there are many digestive system illnesses that occur due to prolonged exposure to improper foods. In a similar vein, most of our skin conditions are signs of diet-caused issues. The list goes on and on. Those are severe warnings that our nutrition is compromising the operation of our bodies.

Despite their incredible resilience, our organs do wear down. In most cases it takes decades of abuse to cause total failure. Until then, they function poorly. There are many symptoms of that impaired operation. We all know them as nuisances that we attribute, for the most part, to the process of aging: We look tired or feel out of sorts; we have a brain-fog or can't sleep or are irritable; we have indigestion or a skin breakout, and so on.

Our digestive system is a biological subsystem that has an optimal operating range. It functions optimally on one daily meal with varying fuels. Currently, we drive our digestion very hard with constant use, and on mostly one kind of fuel: carbohydrates. What can we expect as a result? Precisely what we are seeing now in our society.

Chapter Eleven

The Human Diet

The response to the question of what our diet should be is really not that difficult—that is, if we regard our body as one should perceive a complex, self-regulating system. Namely, interference with the system should be avoided; the best approach is hands-off. Let the system operate naturally. In reference to our body, "natural operation" is the functioning that closely follows our evolutionary adaptation. We should not try to impose the consumption of meals consisting of arbitrarily chosen foods eaten according to a schedule. Instead, we should stick with the variable hunter-gatherer menu consumed when required and not a moment sooner.

After all, we are "optimized" for a sporadic food supply and radical diet switching. That was our way of living for roughly half a million years. Nowadays, however, we have stopped exercising that dietary agility.

Let's compare our modern eating style to our optimal food intake.

Diet	Original	Modern
Food	Mostly Meat Simply Processed	Mostly Plants Heavily Processed
Variety	No Staple From Carnivore to Vegan	Staple: Grain Supplementary Foods Variable
Meals per Day	One	Three with Snacking
Fasting	Intermittent Whole Day Multi-Day Dry	No
Macronutrients	Variable Ratio From Keto through Low-Carb to High-Carb	Steady Ratio High-Carb

From the above table, it's apparent that our modern nutrition is far removed from our genetic adaptation. Searching for the ideal diet focused on fixed macronutrient ratios is an exercise in futility. Most people feel better when changing diets, at least for a while. And it's understandable that specific carb/fat/protein proportions work for some people better than others. To put it simply, depending on how far away from the equator your ancestors ventured, you'll be less adapted to the higher carbohydrate, lower-fat diet. However, one thing we have in common is the necessity of the periodical shift of our sustenance composition across the macronutrient spectrum. That is what our forefathers did, and that seems to be optimal for humans.

All recently proposed diets recommend sticking to certain food groups or macronutrient ratios. In a way, they are all antithetical to the real human diet, as they impose limits on our dietary choices. Our nomadic predecessors couldn't afford to be selective with what they consumed. In order to survive, they had to move between the carnivore and vegan and between the low-carbohydrate and keto way of eating. Radical diet switching was made possible by nutritionally enhancing harvested foods. We aren't omnivores who directly devour animals (in raw meat form) and graze on wild vegetation. Also, being omnivorous was different for our ancestors than what we consider ourselves to be now—adding meat or fish in roughly the same proportion to a starchy staple and swapping similar foods all year round is not what the prototypical *Homo sapiens* did.

We hear the word "moderation" frequently from centenarians when they are asked about their longevity secret. They tell us that they consume their food in moderation and are moderately active. In other words, they strike a balance between engaging their muscles and brain just enough to exercise them periodically, and they eat just enough to compensate for that moderate energy expenditure. What if the ideal utilization of our bodies constitutes exactly that—exercising all our muscles, brain, and the organs related to digestion and metabolism? All in moderation. A shifting of nutrition means exercising various digestive paths one at a time while letting the others rest. Occasional fasting lets the whole body get into recuperation mode. To go with that, we should probably also exercise our long-term energy storage. That means that we should put on a few pounds once in a while and shed them promptly after several months.

Let's look at a way to emulate the *Homo sapiens* diet.

Since there is not much science addressing unconventional eating patterns, we have to rely on logic to evaluate its merits.

Intuitively speaking, while eating one meal a day, the body should be capable of accommodating changes in macronutrient ratios very well. That intuition comes from looking at our ancestors' prolonged adaptation to their wide range of foods. We can fashion our diet shifts the same way our ancestors used to experience. The intention here is to follow the availability of plant foods throughout the year and to replace them with meat and fish in times of vegetation scarcity. Naturally, the warmer months would add more vegetation to the diet, with the summer additions of fruit and grains. The transformation of the menu would go from carb-y in the summer to keto in the dead of winter. It's reasonable to assume that cravings played a significant role for our ancestors as the guiding force in choosing sustenance. After all, there is a reason we desire variability in our meals. And our predecessors had a chance of significantly altering their menu every few months. One can imagine the intense appetite for carbohydrates after a period of high-fat, low-starch diet (and the other way around). That craving throughout the year could have conveniently coincided with seasonal foods' availability.

Hence, summertime would increase the proportion of carbs on the menu. At its peak, the ratio of carbohydrates, protein, and fat would approach the low-fat, high-carbohydrate diet that is prescribed today. It would contain grains, beans, potatoes, a variety of fruit, little meat or fish, and very little fat. To enhance variability, it may make sense to vary the sources of the carbohydrates.

In the spring and fall, we would eat roughly according to the Paleo diet. This means a moderate amount of meat and fish, nuts, seeds, low-sugar fruit, and moderate carbohydrates.

A portion of the winter diet would constitute the low-carbohydrate diet, with a month or two of the keto diet. This means meat, fish, plenty of fat, and minimal to no carbohydrates.

As our ancestors did most of the time, we should attempt to eat only one big meal daily. The feast should be large enough to provide adequate calories for the day. The consolidation of eating is excellent for practical reasons, as it makes controlling the portion size and macronutrient ratios very easy.

In the summer, for a month or two, there could be a broader, few-hours-long feasting window to accommodate the longer day and lower-fat (fewer calories) sustenance.

A diet like this should give our digestive system a chance to cycle through the macronutrient range. Note that a similar nutrient cycling can be achieved by changing the diet on a monthly and weekly basis. In addition, the frequency and range of the changes may be modified to suit the individual. If we want to go further in emulating our ancestors' eating habits, we should add fasting to our routine.

We could abstain from food for variable periods. To follow our ancestors' model, we could have more frequent or longer fasts in the winter and early spring—the reasoning being that those seasons lack the vegetable fallback sustenance.

For people not spending much time outside, which is most of us, the diet should be supplemented with vitamin D. To match our ancestors' vitamin D synthesis, doses of the vitamin should follow the sun and our physical activity.

It's difficult to know how our farming-distorted eating habits affect our health. However, seeing how much modern nutrition diverges from its prototypical model, our constitution might be significantly compromised. The fact that we abuse our digestive system should give us a scare. We use our gastrointestinal tract three times more frequently than our predecessors. Not counting snacking, we eat twenty-one times weekly, while our ancestors would typically do so just seven times. The difference over the course of a decade would be about seven thousand more meals eaten. Despite our all-day feeding, we don't skip any days; we over-engage our digestion steadily all year round, even though we can function without food for extended periods. Imagine how that aspect of our modern diet alone impacts our longevity.

While our omnivorous nature is geared toward using fats, proteins, and carbohydrates as interchangeable primary energy sources, our food production methods generally make us go with the starches. Let's consider the following. Fats contain nine calories per gram, and their digestion costs only zero to three percent of the consumed calories. Carbohydrates, on the other hand, hold only four calories, and their assimilation requires five to ten percent. So, fats are the most efficient and absorbable energy sources. Thus, they are very practical nutrients, despite being not as instantly rewarding to our brains as carbohydrates.

Consequently, using carbs instead of fats to supply the same number of calories, we must ingest more food, thereby putting more stress on our digestive system. Another health problem may be the rigidity of the macronutrient ratio. We don't shift our diet regularly from high- to low-carbohydrate, taking it all the way to keto. The periods of fasting and diet switching are natural and yet considered generally unhealthy by modern nutritional science. Why?

As humans, we possess the potential to modify our surroundings. Unlike other animals, which mostly try to adapt to the environment, we purposefully work to change it to suit our needs. In some cases, we notice that our improvements go too far too fast. For example, we recognize environmental pollution as a negative aspect of our progress. However, regarding nutrition, despite clear warning signs, we cannot admit that we have strayed far from our optimal diet. Is that because this eating transition happened a long time ago?

That fateful change resolved the problem of irregular and nutritionally uneven food supply. Thus we have solved, so it would seem, within a short time, the predicament with which we had struggled for ages along with other animals. As beneficial as that solution was to our civilizational progress, it also had its adverse health consequences, as it has moved us away from our natural food consumption.

Let's look closer at the pre-farming era, the period that distinguished us from the rest of the animal kingdom and shaped us genetically as modern humans. That was the era when, exercising our superior intelligence, we learned to enhance our food and thus made our meals more nutritious and predictable. We skillfully hunted game, extracted the best edible parts of vegetation, and further enhanced them by cooking. Thus, by creating nutritional options, we turned into extreme high-caloric-meal omnivores, radically switching source-foods based on opportunity. Becoming less reliant on our environment, we were capable of roaming over the vast expanses of the planet, unlike any other animal. Less reliant does not mean independent, as at that time our eating habits were still subject to the fluctuations and seasonality imposed by nature. That period was evolutionary viable. And in fact, to this day our bodies remain attuned to the unsteady quality, quantity, and composition of sustenance. That means that periods of calorie restrictions or absence and macronutrient shifts are essential to our health. Regardless of our comfort level, that is our optimal eating environment. For many of us, it's hard to imagine that the unsteadiness of our diet can improve our health; it doesn't seem to make sense in our hyper-organized modern reality. That distorted perception is an example of the collision of messy reality with our liking for order and predictability. Whereas that misperception can be forgiven us as consumers, it can't justify the complacency of the scientists researching these nutritional issues.

Chapter Twelve

Fixing the Diet

The current worldwide food dystopia must end. We have to rethink our untenable attitude toward nutrition. We can't have our cake and eat it too. That is to say, we can't maximize our eating pleasure while staying healthy. That boils down to the question: Should we continue to live to eat or start to eat to live?

Despite a general awareness of junk food, most people don't fully realize the real consequences of unhealthy eating. Conversely, most of us don't grasp the enormous self-healing potential of our bodies when they function according to their evolutionary blueprint. It's the potential with which we are born but which we squander by deviating from our optimal eating path.

We have been on the wrong nutritional track since the start of the farming era. However, modern industrial food production and pricing structure made the situation even worse. We massively and consistently overeat. That overindulgence is not something in which we participate cool-headedly. We are in the midst of a culture obsessed with food. We live in a world focused on eating to an unhealthy degree. This is not a recent phenomenon. We've been building ceremonial, socializing, hedonistic eating values for centuries. The festive aspect of it used to help us bond socially, and it's still useful for that purpose. However, we extended the celebratory character of eating into our daily routine. Unlike in the past, cheap caloric food is easy to come by. Therefore, we overeat daily just because we can. That approach naturally collides with the desire to stay trim and healthy.

In that environment, we move between two extremes—gluttony and dieting. Both of them are unsustainable in the long term. We need to logically and systematically transform our culture of eating.

We can forgive our farmer-ancestors for the menu choices they made. After all, the switch of diet was a practical one, done in the name of progress. With farming based on grain, they were able to feed more people and spur civilizational progress. With the other dominant causes of the short life expectancy at the time, more physical activity and limited grain production, the health issues caused by the dietary shift were barely noticeable. Now, however, the catastrophic state of our health points directly to the traditional farmer's way of eating as the main culprit. Thus, it's inexcusable not to reconsider that millennia-old fateful decision. The question we should ask is, what is the best diet for us? Is it the diet that we invented or the one that we evolved to follow?

For expediency reasons, authorities have decided not to challenge the ten-thousand-year-old choice. Our governing bodies continue to promote the massive consumption of foods that are cheap to manufacture on a large scale. Also, they keep backing the frequent eating schedule as the healthiest way to eat. However, did anybody do the math regarding the full cost of making us "happy" with the massive flow of cheap, super-caloric foods? It's like buying a car and looking only at the sticker price while ignoring the cost of ownership. If the car is shiny and inexpensive but keeps breaking down, and the cost of repairs is exorbitant, is the purchase still a bargain? Our affordable, tasty, and massively consumed food is not a good deal. When we add to its cost the expense of our bodily "maintenance," we may well conclude that our nourishment is very pricey. In fact, our budget is caving in under the weight of healthcare expenses. Still, putting aside the monetary considerations, we lose something that is unquantifiable—our well-being.

As long as our personal and historical recollections reach into the past, the starchy staples in our three daily meals indicated prosperity and comfort. Maybe the current enormous health crisis will motivate us to change that. The stakes couldn't be any higher.

So where do we go from here? Is there a practical way out of our infatuation with food? What can be done to move us away from the addictive, harmful diet of our creation toward the proper human food consumption model?

The first step is to modify the pleasure/comfort attitude toward eating. Everybody must realize that the principal purpose of eating is very pedestrian. It's to provide the best nutrients necessary for our active lives and long-term health. It's not to give us maximal eating pleasure—at least, not all the time. Ten thousand years ago, the sense of taste used to guide us toward better nutrition. Farming and food processing, including elaborate cooking, changed that. We shifted the balance of flavor to a degree way beyond what our ancestors were used to. To realize our full health potential, we should, for the most part, stay within the Stone Age eating schedule and menu shifts. However, since our foods are totally different, we shouldn't overthink our specific food choices. Eating for pleasure can have its place—but it should be occasional and fully informed.

A real nutritional transformation can only take place when we change the social attitude toward pleasure eating. That can be done in the same way we changed our perception of smoking. What we accomplished there was deglamorizing tobacco use. In the same vein, we have to show the real consequences of eating as a diversion. Smoking and eating for pleasure are more alike than we care to admit. They are both harmful, highly addictive, and unnecessary. However, while most of us were outraged at the tobacco companies for adding extra nicotine to their cigarettes, we never noticed that we spiked our foods by deep-frying them, added excessive salt and sugar, and otherwise "improved" their taste to make them quasi-narcotics. And still, we recommend eating them steadily throughout the day.

In their entertainment role, foods are very similar to alcohol and recreational drugs. One difference is that alcohol and drug consumption undergoes strict social and legal scrutiny. Another one, which makes our attitude toward food so ambivalent, is that food is, unlike drugs, also a life-supporting necessity. That duality of function as both the source of pleasure and an imperative of survival is very confusing.

I propose some practical steps we can take toward nutritional emancipation:

Sugar and sweetened food prices should be raised. That could be achieved by adding a tax to sweetened foods proportionally to their sugar content. This sugar tax, implemented gradually over the span of a few years, would give us and the industry time to adjust.

A campaign should be launched to inform consumers about the harmful effects of the frequent consumption of celebratory foods.

The recommended three meals daily should be replaced with "eat and drink when hungry and thirsty" advice, which boils down to one meal daily (or a short daily eating period).

Occasional fasting should be encouraged.

Diet recommendations should be rewritten. The varying macronutrient ratio should be officially advised. Specific fruit, grain, and dairy recommendations should be removed. There should be strong warnings about the harmful nature of sugar and the addictive properties of dairy and the carbohydrate/fat combination.

Food labels must be simplified. They should contain indicators of how a given food compares to others regarding the essential characteristics which affect our health. For example, as mentioned in this book, fiber density and carbohydrate content would be helpful in plant-based food products, plus color-coding to allow for quickly discerning the nutritional and potentially addictive properties of food items.

Authorities should start working on restructuring our food production to align it with the goal of feeding the population with more varied foods and producing it in a more environmentally friendly and sustainable manner.

Vitamin D should be an officially recommended supplement, and the dietary correction for children should be put in place to prevent our current widespread orthodontic problems.

And finally, intensive food-industry-independent research should be carried out on the subject of the human genetically aligned diet.

Chapter Thirteen

My Human Diet Experience

Up until a few years ago, I did not pay much attention to nutrition. Of course, I was aware of the widespread overeating problem. However, as is the case with many, I was under the impression that the so-called junk food served by fast food restaurants was the sole (or at least primary) offender. I thought that eating home-cooked meals was the way to stay healthy. Since I rarely patronized fast food establishments, I considered myself a healthy eater. Sure, I was carrying a few extra pounds, but I was comforted by thinking I was not outside the norm. Even during my annual checkups, I wasn't admonished for my extra poundage. I guess that with my six-foot-two frame, the twenty to thirty extra pounds were not that apparent. When I was younger, I was able to shed the extra pounds when I wanted to, and I did that occasionally. However, as I got older, I was so wrapped up in everyday life that I just stopped thinking about the pouch I was carrying around. And as the years went by, it was more and more difficult to let go of my favorite foods. Like most people, I loved my rich foods. The common theme among them was high carbohydrate content combined with fat. I enjoyed that butter spread on potatoes and dipping my pizza in melted garlic butter. Sweets, too, were near the top of my favorites list. Curiously, I was able to stop adding sugar to my tea and coffee.

Also, I didn't like my desserts too sweet; it felt like the excess sugar prevented me from enjoying larger portions of the treats.

Therefore, I wasn't a big fan of very sweet cakes and candy. Not to the degree that I would refuse one, mind you, but sweets weren't my first choice. No, I loved balance in my desserts—enough of the creamy fats juxtaposed with some proteins and that perfect measure of sweetness. I just couldn't resist that sublime blend of all three macronutrients. Ice cream always did it for me. My favorite flavors were butter pecan and pistachio. There is something about the nature-balanced milk, eggs, and nuts with a little sugar blended in for that extra enticement. Remarkably, most of the mass market ice cream producers discovered how to formulate their products to achieve that exact balance of taste. Their marketing department must have figured that out as a secret to maximizing sales: Don't oversweeten the product but leave it a bit less intense in order to tempt the customer to eat much more of it. That's pure genius!

I've got to admit that ice cream, either in a cone as a daily treat or topped with chocolate fudge, extra nuts, and whipped cream on the weekend is impossible for me to resist. Yes, I am a sugarholic. But from comparing myself to friends and acquaintances, I can tell that I am not an extreme one. Many people can't let go of the taste of sweetness, even in their drinks. They sweeten their coffee and tea and wash down their meals with soda, on top of consuming their sugar in cereals, condiments, and desserts. Although I can drink water and unsweetened hot drinks, the power of attraction that ice cream exerts on me is unbelievably strong. I don't hesitate to call that pull what it is: an addiction. As a former smoker, I can compare how ice cream and cigarettes used to control my brain. When I was obeying those cravings, that is, smoked regularly or consumed my ice cream on a daily basis, my world was fine; I wasn't aware of my dependence. In the case of tobacco, I was just being cool like other grownups (that was in the times of the common acceptance of tobacco use). As to the ice cream, frequent indulgence just felt like a food preference. However, in both cases, when I tried to stop, I would go through the similar addiction-characteristic head games. I would think along the lines of: "It's not a big deal; one will not harm me," or "Just another one and then I stop," or "I deserve it after my hard day of work." Somehow the relinquishing of my favorite snack grew in my mind to the magnitude of a humongous sacrifice. I must say that the cigarette addiction was stronger for me than the ice cream one. However, sugar dependence is very tricky, as it can move from one sweet food to another. Thus, when I was trying to quit ice cream, I would "escape" to pancakes soaked in syrup, cereals, or various fruits. Fruits, in particular, made me feel much better about myself. I even used them sometimes as a meal replacement. So at times, after wolfing down my fifth banana, I felt that I was on the right nutritional track. As with sugar, other carbohydrates also make us jump between the amazingly "satisfying" foods. For years, a solid portion of carbs accompanied my every meal. There was no exception; breakfast, lunch, and dinner came with bread, pasta, rice, or potatoes. However, as carb-y as my meals were, I was shocked to discover that some people double up on their carbs. For example, it's common for Italians to eat their bread with pasta!

My nutritional ups and downs gave me some food for thought. However, the firsthand observation of how easy it is to combat a serious illness with nutrition startled me. My mom's amazing, easy recovery from diabetes gave me the final push to write this book. My mom is eighty-two. For many years she was overweight and suffered from diabetes type two and the accompanying heart problems. She had always loved to cook and indulge in sumptuous meals. She used to eat a variety of them. On the menu were starches in the form of pasta and potatoes; meats including poultry, beef, and occasionally pork, with ribs being her favorite; and fish like tuna, salmon, and the occasional lobster. She always had veggies to accompany dinner. Fruit and dairy were popular in her house. She rarely ate out and even more rarely ate junk food. However, she loved sweets, especially various fruits or ice cream for dessert. She cooked her meals and made sure to eat veggies and fruit every day. Under that routine, she had been struggling with her weight since her early forties. Of course, being overweight, her mobility was limited. She wasn't very active and was naturally very unhappy about it.

After my stepfather passed away, I started taking care of my mom. That included grocery shopping for her. Knowing about her health problems, I convinced her to start changing her diet. One by one, I stopped buying her favorite calorie bombs. First I stopped getting her ice cream and chocolates. Then I brought more greens to replace some of the starches.

The change in her diet boiled down to replacing rich meals with salads. I changed her menu over the period of a few months. Then I convinced her to change the times of her meals. Instead of breakfast at eight, lunch at noon, and dinner at five, she switched to just lunch at noon and dinner at four.

Curiously, she doesn't miss her hearty starches with fats. She smoothly transitioned to salads. A significant reason for the painless menu change is that she isn't exposed to external temptations. She lives alone and I deliver her groceries. The base of her salads consists of avocado, broccoli, and tomato with occasional lettuce and onion. She makes the salad in two bowls before noon. She eats the salads with chicken, tuna, or hard-boiled eggs with a dab of mayo. On the side, she has a piece of whole bread with butter and smoked salmon. She usually eats only one piece of bread a day—half a slice with each meal. Every few weeks she swaps the bread for beans.

After four months of the salad diet, we went to her doctor

for a checkup. Her weight had dropped by thirty pounds and all her diabetes markers had gone back to normal. If I had any doubts about the role diet plays in our lives, I had proof in front of me. At the age of eighty-two, without exercising, one can easily reverse a serious health condition just by changing one's way of eating. While that is pretty obvious to many people, I don't think most of us realize the full impact of what it means. For me, it means that it's impossible to underestimate the importance of foods and the way we eat them. It's the absolute key to our well-being.

As I aged, I started having annoying little health problems. I was often tired during the day, had occasional stomach discomfort and headaches, couldn't sleep at night, and my skin was either too oily or too dry. All those complaints, when mentioned to physicians, were deflected by directing me to over-the-counter remedies. At first, I just accepted that advice and used the ointments, digestive aids, and sleeping pills as directed. However, those measures, assisted with increased doses of caffeine, didn't work very well. I just felt "blah" throughout the day, with little energy and frequent mental fog. The nights were not much better, as I would frequently have trouble falling asleep and wake up in the night.

It took me years to start looking around for alternative solutions. When I did, even rudimentary research made me aware of just how many people are in the same boat. There are a huge number of them living with similar marginal health problems—and a myriad of ways they try to cope. One of them is trying to find a missing nutrient. Following the supplementation-as-a-remedy path, I have built quite a stockpile of supplements, trying in vain to find the right combination. As I reflect on it now, I see how fallacious my thinking was. I was naively trying to add a missing ingredient to my diet, something that I can't absorb from food or that my body is unable to synthesize on its own. As if I were likely to stumble on one among the huge numbers of compounds which may be responsible for my symptoms and through pure luck achieve better results than trained people in research labs all over the world have been able to do. I see the self-medication attempts differently now—as an act of desperation on our part, like betting on new sets of compounds and believing our luck will change with another delivery of health boosters in the mail.

That search for a lacking supplement is a very common quest which makes sense to us intuitively because it is bolstered by the media serving us stories that describe the amazing powers of this or that food or compound. Those exaggerated anecdotes about magic berries, mushrooms, or algae are just that. Most of them have some micro-dose of truth in them, but their efficacy is inflated more and more as the story is retold. We are conditioned to look for simple solutions and we are offered simplistic pseudo-truths as answers.

I must admit that I had bitten the bait. I went down the rabbit hole of supplementation and magic foods wholeheartedly. I also tried different diets. For about a year I tried the low-carbohydrate diet and I felt significantly better while on it; however, eating the obligatory three meals, I still had a hard time controlling my weight. Of all my dietary experiments, the most interesting was fasting. When I tried it, I experienced a significant difference in the way I felt. At first, the empty stomach made me feel uncomfortable. Not physically, but mentally. I thought I was sacrificing something by not having my breakfast and lunch, as I wasn't used to having my belly completely empty. But over time, the daily fasting made me realize that it's the state I *should* be in. Without food in my stomach, I operated at a completely different level, both physically and mentally. I recognized how digestion slowed me down. Skipping meals made me feel better, regardless of the carbohydrate content of my menu. However, lowering the carbohydrates in combination with eating once daily was where the magic happened for me. And I mean magic.

After only a few weeks of having only one low- to moderate-carbohydrate meal a day, my body started to change. The most significant differences were in my skin. My dermatological issues—dryness, roughness, puffiness around the eyes, and skin discolorations—began disappearing. I could also smell the difference. Even after exercising, my sweat seemed to be neutral; there was no discernible smell to it, as if my body chemistry had changed. My muscles started looking more defined with the same level of exercise, indicating a rise in testosterone level.

Interestingly, the efficiency of my body's food utilization increased. For my one meal, I was naturally eating more than the equivalent portion of one of my previous meals. However, the difference was not that significant. I ate between a quarter and three quarters more than the amount of food that used to constitute my dinner. It has taken me a while to figure out the appropriate portion size. In the beginning, I was continually overeating, as I mistakenly thought that I had to be close with my calorie intake to the combined three-meals-daily figure. Therefore, I had been packing in extra food at the end of the meal, afraid of precipitous weight loss. However, by eating more substantial meals, my weight went up. Seeing that, I gradually reduced the portion to a more reasonable size. With only one meal to consider, my weight control became easy. To lose weight, I just decreased my food intake slightly. Conversely, I would overeat somewhat to gain weight. The astonishing fact for me is that by eating one meal daily I was consuming much less food without being hungry and losing weight, but with better cognitive and physical functioning. It seems that on the human diet digestion and metabolism work differently than on the farmer's diet. I believe that the fasted state-induced hormonal/

metabolic shift is responsible for the more efficient extraction and utilization of energy from food.

At first, dropping my breakfast and lunch wasn't a pleasant experience. I felt a little deprived in the afternoon, as the anticipation of dinner frequently preoccupied my thoughts.

In time, however, the between-meal period started to become more natural. I stopped feeling uneasy about the empty stomach. Instead, I felt more comfortable without eating and thinking about the next feeding. There were days when I was so busy that I would skip my one meal altogether. The place of eating in my hierarchy of importance slipped from the foreground to the background. When I wasn't hungry, there were more important things to do than eating, exactly like when I was a kid. I didn't set a fixed mealtime. I figured that I should control my feeding by varying the quantity of food rather than the time of the meal. That way I wouldn't have to be distracted too much by hunger. If one day my hunger manifested early, I would obey it. For my earlier meal, I typically ate more so that the next day I would just go back to the usual 5:00 p.m. mealtime.

After about three months on the human diet, my cravings subsided. I lost thirty pounds with minimal exercise. My muscles grew significantly and my energy increased. After the initial low-carb period, I felt confident enough to start varying my carbohydrate content. I noticed that after a few months of lower starch intake, increasing it is quite uneventful. Unlike previously, I don't feel the ill effects of their occasionally higher concentration. However, keeping in mind my prior experiences, I am careful about keeping the carb-y days adequately spaced.

Unsurprisingly, one meal daily makes me enjoy eating more than before. And, switching between different carb ratios is much less noticeable. Thus the transition from a more starchy meal one day to a salad the next doesn't feel like much of a sacrifice. It looks like hunger, even a mild one, is the big craving equalizer. As hard as it is to imagine eating salads for breakfast, lunch, and dinner, it's natural for me to consume them once a day for a few days in a row.

The following are my thoughts on the human diet in our modern reality.

Apart from processing our food, we are like all other mammals. As such, we should be attuned to our body, as it will give us signals about when to eat and drink. But we must be vigilant about the ingredients we crave most. Those are typically beneficial for us when consumed in moderation since they used to be rare in our natural environment.

As modern people, instead of being partially at the mercy of nature when it comes to food choices, we are in total control.

I understand that practically all our foods are refined to a certain degree. They are different from the foods available in the wild. That refinement happens either through farming or industrial processing. However, the fact that we don't eat raw foods is not a reason to panic. Actually, it's quite convenient. Our ancestors had to work hard to adapt their wild foods for consumptions. They were usually processing their foods daily.

We don't. We can create our meals easily with the desired balance of nutrients and fiber. However, as we know, there is a difference between processed and overprocessed foods. For example, the farmed vegetables that we can consume directly are technically refined from their wild counterpart. Therefore, we can eat them in their raw or cooked form without much concern.

Sugar and white flour, on the other hand, are way overprocessed for our digestion, as is most of our cultivated fruit. We have to keep in mind that in nature, even moderately dense carbohydrate and fat sources were quite rare. Therefore, a higher concentration of those ingredients in our meals should raise a red flag.

[125]

On the other hand, we eat meals, not individual foods. Thus, as long as the meal has a proper ingredient balance, the individual foods don't really matter that much. An occasional fruit, potato, or piece of bread accompanied by veggies should be okay.

This is how I look at balancing my meals: I pay close attention to varying the macronutrient ratios. The vitamin and mineral consumption takes care of itself when I frequently consume salads, meats, and nuts. I use salads to dilute the carbohydrate content and nuts to add fats and easily boost my calorie intake. With this method, it's easy to effectively vary my daily meal's composition.

The most important part of the human diet is not to eat more than once a day or eat only within the range of a few short hours. That, for me, kills the cravings. When I am finally ready for a meal, I eat with a similar enthusiasm no matter what's on the table. And I don't fear an occasional piece of bread or even a sweet addition to my meal once in a while.

Overall, I think that it's not that hard to function nowadays eating according to a proper human diet. Even accommodating a social situation may be possible without attracting too much attention. When I go to a function requiring me to participate in a meal, I just fast before it. Dinners are more convenient, as they agree better with my eating schedule. Now, since I learned to ignore the mild hunger that sometimes occurs when I shift my eating schedule, even breakfasts and lunches are okay for me. Of course, my meal is usually larger than everybody else's. It's kind of amusing when you're quite slim and devour more food than anybody else at the table. They all assume that you have a better metabolism. And in a way that's true.

My view is that trying to eat one meal daily doesn't mean that it's a great transgression to eat two or even three meals a day occasionally. As long as it doesn't become a rule, I consider those deviations as a part of exercising my eating flexibility.

I would like to mention a few changes I've noticed when eating one meal daily with varied macronutrient ratio. The first of those is a completely different perception of hunger. Since my late twenties, I have reacted badly to skipping a meal; usually, after a few hours past my mealtime, I would develop a pounding headache or I would become very irritable. The anticipation of that unpleasant reaction of my body had been keeping me very conscious of my meal schedule. When I switched to one meal daily, I still reacted that way for a while. Not every day, but once in a while during the first month, I would have those occasional off days. However, my feeling of hunger diminished significantly with time, as did that of thirst. But my tiredness after the meal is more pronounced than that occurring after one of three daily meals. As alert as my mind is now on an empty stomach, for a few hours after my meal, I feel as if I have taken a tranquilizer. Not surprisingly, perhaps, my restroom schedule also underwent changes during my diet transition. Without going into the details, I never go to bed feeling full now.

Nevertheless, the changes my body experienced after just a few months were quite significant. Now I understand much better the distinction between digestion/rest and fasted/active states. And I realize that through the farmer's diet we banish our natural metabolic state from our waking hours.

Conclusion

We can't fully realize our health potential until we fix that pivotal aspect of our life, our diet. Until we do, we can't tell which anomalies are related to nutrition and which are due to hereditary or external influences. Consider this: Even our gene expression may depend on the diet. So, the correlation we discover between certain gene sequences and serious health conditions may be valid only because of our unnatural way of eating.

However, based on those predictions, many people reach for extreme measures to avoid the dreaded deadly diseases that are foretold by their genetics.

We have a certain bias in the perception of our bodies' wellness potential. We see people around us plagued with various health issues, from bad teeth and skin rashes to digestive problems, to severe heart conditions and cancers. We notice pharmacies on every street corner and the steady stream of ads promoting medications, doctors, and hospitals. Based on that exposure, we intuitively assume that our common afflictions are to be expected in the grand scheme of things. We assume it is typical that our bodies start unraveling from the age of about 30 to be just barely functioning by our mid-60s. We accept that the vast majority of people over 65 must suffer from one or more severe health issues. Those expectations are based on our current reality and fully warranted. However, we need to realize that the health issues we experience may be related to the fact that we as a society are not following the proper human diet.

A nutritional rewind to the times of the hunter-gatherer has already been proposed in the context of the Paleo Diet—and the idea has faced opposition from many nutritionists, whose arguments range from reasonable to ridiculous. One of the seemingly reasonable arguments is that most of the available plant foods we eat are not the same as they used to be before farming; another is that there was no single diet for all humans, as they ate different foods depending on geographical location. Another source of quibbling comes from considering the human digestive system, a factor used against as well as for many other specific diets: People who argue for vegetarianism say our intestines are too long for carnivorous eating, while meat proponents say they are too short for vegetarian eating.

Let's consider those opinions. They sound reasonable based on the assumption that humans eat their food raw. That presumption, however, flies in the face of the main message of this book—the significance of our food preparation. Our digestive system is the size that it is because it is perfectly optimized for *processed* meat and plants. Our optimal nutrition, therefore, consists of foods that are refined and otherwise prepared for our digestion. As long as their nutrient levels fall within a certain optimal range, the kind of food is not that important.

The meat we eat isn't raw, so comparing humans to lions and tigers doesn't make any sense. By the same token, comparing us to antelopes and cows is ridiculous. Even lumping us together with other omnivores that feed on raw meat and plants is not entirely accurate; although we are technically omnivores, we don't eat our foods raw, as they do. We mostly eat meals of our own creation which aren't available in nature. We use a wide range of sources, both plants and animals, to create our sustenance.

As discussed previously, food treatment has been the hallmark of our species since the dawn of humanity. We evolved out of the realm of the raw-eaters a long time ago—hence our relatively small teeth and fragile stomachs. Through skillful food preparation, we have become much less dependent on specific plant and animal sources. However, most of today's nutritional approaches are fixated on particular foods, specific macronutrient ratios, and nutrients (or lack thereof). Those factors, while relevant, are secondary to eating frequency and the need to vary our meals' macronutrient structure.

Eating only once per day, as humans used to do, puts significant brakes on overeating by stabilizing cravings and physically limiting calorie intake. Additionally, the nearly 24-hour periods between meals bring about the powerful healing benefits of fasting. Occasional multiday fasts amplify that thorough recuperation mode.

In conjunction with that approach, varying fat and carbohydrate concentration in our meals should rectify our intestinal microbial imbalance. A healthy gut then strengthens the immune system as well as the nervous system, as the state of our digestive system significantly influences our brain. Our body has a powerful gut-brain connection; our digestive system impacts our physical, behavioral, and emotional brain functions. Thus, the health benefits of conforming to our primal nutritional adaptation could be enormous.

Ironically, the science behind the human diet is sketchy. However, the results of studies dealing with some of the aspects of this diet, like fasting and ketosis, are very promising. The list of the health benefits suggested by those studies is very long and sounds almost too good to be true. It mentions, among others, slowing down the aging process, dramatically reducing the risks of many serious illnesses, and improving our cognitive and physical functions.

Now, let's think about this for a moment. How surprising is it that the way of eating we evolved into is great for us? I would say hardly. After all, it's our optimal diet. However, our general disinterest regarding the inappropriateness of our currently promoted unnatural nutrition is quite startling.

Only after we begin eating like *Homo sapiens* ought to can we consider other flaws of modern nutrition, like overprocessed foods, chemical food additives, and foods that provide inadequate fiber, vitamin, and mineral intake. Focusing on those issues while on our current artificial farmer's diet is putting the cart in front of the horse.

We shouldn't be scared of modern foods. Considering, of course, that we need to mind the overprocessed ones, we can be glad that we may walk into the store and pick from a variety of comestibles suitable for human consumption. We don't have to go outside and pick berries and nuts or hunt antelope to comply with the essence of our nutritional adaptation, as we have at our disposal a conveniently prepared cornucopia of foods. Our modern vegetables, for example, are nontoxic, have the right amount of fiber, and are very easy to prepare. Bread, potatoes, or even fruit combined with a salad or consumed on our high-carbohydrate days shouldn't be a problem. Even infrequent fast food consumption shouldn't scare us; remember that we have evolved to accommodate an occasional overindulgence.

Transitioning to our primal diet should probably make us reconsider our current attitudes toward hygiene, including the use of soaps and body care cosmetics. To put it simply, our prototypical body care makes sense, as it was associated for millennia with our ancestral nomadic diet.

To follow in their footsteps, we may get some cues from the simplicity of the hygienic routine of our nomadic forefathers. While we may not want to completely abandon washing our bodies and brushing our teeth, we may take a critical look at our everyday bathing and use of soaps, shampoos, lotions, tonics, and creams. As discussed earlier in this book, our bodies are adept at balancing their microbiota.

Similarly to treating the microbes in our digestive system, we should provide the microorganisms on our skin the optimal conditions to thrive. Like our GI tract, our skin constitutes a barrier between our body and the external environment. Therefore, it's very important that this large, active boundary has optimal conditions to fully realize its defensive properties. For hundreds of thousands of years, our Stone Age forefathers' skin auto-regulated its chemistry with specific bodily secretions, the composition of which favored certain types of microbes while suppressing proliferation of others. That distinct composition of our body's "cultivated" microbiota is what's optimal for our skin. Our nomadic ancestors didn't use soap. They most likely just washed their skin occasionally with water.

We know that interference with the microbiota can have serious consequences. For example, the presence of antibiotics or lack of fiber in our GI tracts may cause severe malfunctioning of our digestion. However, similarly to indiscriminately killing off bacteria with antibiotics in our digestive system, we routinely get rid of the microbial colonies on our skin by frequently washing our bodies with soap. The right composition of skin microbes constitutes a vital part of our skin's external defensive shield. Getting rid of that carefully balanced colony can make it easier for hostile microbes to invade our body.

The proper inhabitants of our skin, in addition to blocking invasions, specialize in breaking down our skin secretions and dead, discarded fragments of our dermis in the best possible way. Now, contrast that sophisticated, mutually beneficial relationship with our attempts at removing our helpers forcibly with soaps and tonics. Add to this picture the application of various lotions and creams that clog skin pores and hamper the rebound of our friendly micro-residents' colonies, and you'll understand that our hygienic/cosmetic interference may be quite harmful.

Skin is our largest organ, and its importance to our general health can't be overstated. Its optimal functioning can be achieved by eating a proper diet and maintaining it the way our ancestors did for countless generations—washing it infrequently with water. Of course, in modern reality, knowing what we know about communicable diseases, we may have to modify that approach accordingly. Namely, we may want to continue washing thoroughly our hands, as they come in contact with our not-always-hygienic environment. However, we should stay clear of chemistry-supported body care routines, including frequent full-body washes.

While I suspect there is significant pressure from various industries to preserve the nutritional status quo, I don't believe it's the foremost factor in our dietary predicament. In my view, the root of our problem is our long-standing eating tradition. The tradition is so cultivated, refined, and revered that it feels right—and it's so ingrained in our culture that it can't be dislodged, even with science.

To a degree, we still live in nutritional antiquity. Our modern diet evolved from prehistory following improving methods of food production. Still, its basic structure is practically the same. Thus, in time-honored tradition, those three daily meals with bread, potatoes, or rice are almost sacred. But that diet strays too far from *Homo sapiens'* natural way of eating to be a viable option for the future. This is especially true now when, despite our medical sophistication, our collective health is severely compromised. At a time when many of us live with diet-diminished life quality and skyrocketing medical care costs, we have a choice: Continue on our current dietary path and cope with the dire consequences, or opt for a change. As uncomfortable as it may be in the short term, in order to thrive we must break with current eating practices and return to the human diet.

About the Author

"The people with ideas have no power and the people with power have no ideas..."
—Harmon Okinyo

Gregory Stypko was born in Gdansk, Poland, and was privileged to witness firsthand the birth of the Solidarity movement in the city in 1980, led by Lech Wałęsa. During that period, Gregory was interned by the communist authorities as an untrustworthy citizen.

Following graduation from the Technical University of Gdansk with a degree in Hydro Acoustics, Gregory emigrated to the United States. There, he has worked as a hardware and software engineer for startups and established corporations in various engineering and managerial roles. He lives with his girlfriend and their dog near the Jersey Shore.

When he has time to himself, Gregory enjoys reading or listening to books; he is fascinated by quantum physics and astrophysics. He has an interest in history, with a particular curiosity about ancient Rome and the late 19th and early 20th centuries.

Gregory also loves sports, is learning to play the piano and is always trying to improve his knowledge of other languages, including French and German, in which he regularly gets his news.

Gregory has always appreciated "out-of-the-box" thinking and the power of ideas. He has written for a low-carb food blog in the past.

You can contact Gregory Stypko at gregstypko@gmail.com.

Citations

[1] U.S. Department of Health and Human Services and U.S. Department of Agriculture. **"2015–2020 Dietary Guidelines for Americans."** 8th Edition. Last modified December 2015.
Accessed March 10, 2018.
https://health.gov/dietaryguidelines/2015/guidelines/.

[2] **"List of the largest fast food restaurant chains."** *Wikipedia.*
Accessed October 3, 2018. **https://en.wikipedia.org/wiki/List_of_the_largest_fast_food_restaurant_chains**.

[3] U.S. Department of Agriculture. **"The Food Supply and Dietary Fiber: Its Availability and Effect on Health. Nutrition Insight 36."**
Accessed October 3, 2018. **https://www.cnpp.usda.gov/sites/default/files/nutrition_insights_uploads/Insight36.pdf**.

[4] National Center for Biotechnology Information (NCBI). **"Health benefits of dietary fiber."**
Accessed October 3, 2018.
https://www.ncbi.nlm.nih.gov/pubmed/19335713.

[5] U.S. Department of Agriculture Economic Research Service. **"A Look at Calorie Sources in the American Diet"** from chart: "Seventy percent of Americans' calories in 2010 were from plant-based foods."
Accessed October 3, 2018.
https://www.ers.usda.gov/amber-waves/2016/december/a-look-at-calorie-sources-in-the-american-diet/.

[6] Cordain, L., S.B. Eaton, J.B. Miller, and K. Hill. **"The paradoxical nature of hunter-gatherer diets: meat-based, yet non-atherogenic."** *PubMed.* Eur J Clin Nutr., March 2002, 56 Suppl1: S42-52.
Accessed October 3, 2018.
https://www.ncbi.nlm.nih.gov/pubmed/11965522.

[7] Manore, M.M. **"Exercise and the Institute of Medicine recommendations for nutrition."** *PubMed.* Curr Sports Med Rep., August 4, 2005 (4):193-8.
Accessed October 3, 2018.
https://www.ncbi.nlm.nih.gov/pubmed/16004827.

[8] **"Western pattern diet."** *Wikipedia.*
Accessed October 3, 2018.
https://en.wikipedia.org/wiki/Western_pattern_diet.

[9] **"Fasting."** *Wikipedia.*
Accessed October 3, 2018.
https://en.wikipedia.org/wiki/Fasting.

[10] **"Autophagy."** *Wikipedia.*
Accessed October 7, 2018.
https://en.wikipedia.org/wiki/Autophagy.

[11] **"Autophagy."** *Wikipedia.*
Accessed October 3, 2018.
https://en.wikipedia.org/wiki/Autophagy#Caloric_restriction.

All the citations in this book are from publicly available resources. Wikipedia quotes are used occasionally as a starting point for discussing certain subjects. Although the public encyclopedia is not the most authoritative source on advanced or controversial topics, it is a consensus-driven, solid reference for common, indisputable ones.

www.ingramcontent.com/pod-product-compliance
Lightning Source LLC
Chambersburg PA
CBHW060609200326
41521CB00007B/711